LOW RESOLUTION BRAIN ELECTROMAGNETIC TOMOGRAPHY
(LORETA)

Basic Concepts and Clinical Applications

This work is dedicated to my daughter, Avery and son, Jackson.
Daddy will have some time to play now -
thank you both for your patience, love and understanding.

LOW RESOLUTION BRAIN ELECTROMAGNETIC TOMOGRAPHY

(LORETA)

Basic Concepts and Clinical Applications

Rex L. Cannon, PhD

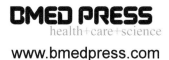

BMED PRESS
health+care+science

www.bmedpress.com

For information about this book:

BMED PRESS
health+care+science

BMED Press, LLC
5656 South Staples St., Suite 302
Corpus Christi, Texas 78411
Phone: (817) 400-1639
www.bmedpress.com

Printed in the United States of America

Cover Design and Layout: Cynthia Kerson, PhD

ISBN-10: 0982749813
ISBN-13: 978-0-9827498-1-4

CONTENTS

LIST OF ILLUSTRATIONS

BMED Press and Rex Cannon, PhD want to express our sincere gratitude to Roberto Pascual-Marqui for his work with LORETA / sLORETA as well as his willingness to freely share these programs with healthcare professionals. We also want to extend a warm 'thank you" for his willingness to grant permission for the use of all LORETA / sLORETA images and figures in this book. We want to further recognize his important and tireless dedication to the advancement of brain science.

Unless otherwise stated, all LORETA / sLORETA figures and images are credited to:

Pascual-Marqui, R. D., Michel, C. M. & Lehmann, D. (1994). Low resolution electromagnetic tomography: a new method for localizing electrical activity in the brain. *Int. J. Psychophysiol.* (18): 4 - 65.

Pascual-Marqui, R.D. (2002). Standardized low-resolution brain electromagnetic tomography (sLORETA): Technical details. *Methods Find Exp Clin Pharmacol 24* (Suppl D): 5 - 12

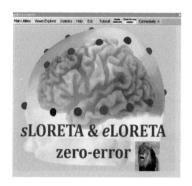

FOREWORD

By Joel F. Lubar, PhD

It is with great pleasure that I am able to write this introduction to Dr. Rex Cannon's volume on LORETA. Our laboratory at the University of Tennessee Knoxville was the first place to develop and utilize LORETA neurofeedback. Our initial publication on this technique was published in 2004. Since that time Dr. Cannon has written and published almost 20 papers on applications of LORETA and LORETA neurofeedback covering areas such as attentional disorders, addiction, and various aspects of memory and more. All of his very impressive publications are listed at the end of this volume. This book is written for both beginners as well as those who are somewhat familiar with the LORETA literature. There is excellent cross validation of LORETA with PET and fMRI.

In the introductory portion of the book there is a clear description of the different EEG frequency bands and their relationship to behavior. Dr. Cannon has pointed out that LORETA is very sensitive to artifacts such as muscle and eye movement and provides excellent examples of how LORETA images are distorted when these artifacts are not eliminated. There are presently three different ways of analyzing LORETA: conventional LORETA involving 2,394 voxels of 7 x 7 x 7 mm, sLORETA, and eLORETA which involves nearly 6,400 voxels of 5 x 5 x 5 mm. The Key Institute programs developed by Dr. Roberto Pascual-Marquis and his colleagues in Zürich allow one in a step-by-step process to convert EEG text files into two and three-dimensional LORETA images involving these three programs. Dr. Cannon takes the reader through the various screens and illustrates procedures for generating these complex images.

This book also contains numerous examples and case studies utilizing LORETA neurofeedback showing both the protocol set up and learning curves that are generated. Currently individuals who are using LORETA neurofeedback are finding that learning is quite rapid especially when using the newer techniques based on Z scores in conjunction with Neuroguide. Since this latter technique involves training different Brodmann areas it is useful to know how these areas differ functionally. This book provides a very detailed coverage of the different Brodmann areas and their functions.

In summary, Dr. Cannon's book brings together important information on LORETA, its development, its applications and potential for the future. This is a very scholarly presentation including nearly 75 pages of references allowing the reader to explore in great detail this extremely valuable approach for understanding human brain function.

An Important Message To Our Readers

The information provided in this book is not a substitute for professional medical or psychological advice or treatment. Always seek the advice of your physician or other qualified health care provider with any questions you may have regarding a medical condition. Always seek the advice of your physician, psychologist, or other qualified healthcare provider with any questions you may have regarding a psychological condition. Never disregard medical or psychological advice or delay in seeking it because of something you have read in this book.

PREFACE

This book was written to provide a method for using LORETA and sLORETA EEG source localization software packages. More importantly, it provides fundamental knowledge of EEG frequency domains and research from other neuroimaging techniques in order to facilitate dissemination of results obtained in this software. This book covers many of the features in the LORETA Key packages while others will be added with time. It is my desire to facilitate the use of LORETA in such a way as to enhance its usability to increase our knowledge of EEG frequency domain functions.

The first portion of the book is dedicated to the use of the LORETA algorithm and components within the LORETA software, including the EEG conversion, transformation matrix, cross spectra, LORETA viewer and statistical tests available to analyze data. The second part covers quantitative EEG, LORETA, and related clinical and experimental data to enhance the experience of the user in designing experiments and to provide rationale for using LORETA. Third, I cover neuroanatomy, Brodmann areas, and the default network of the brain. Finally, ethical and theoretical notions are discussed.

In my early experience of learning EEG and LORETA, I often found myself searching thousands of research articles to describe the outcomes of both simple experiments and complex neurofeedback paradigms. Thus, it was my goal to provide such mechanism to facilitate the use of LORETA and provide a large empirical neuroimaging base from which to interpret the data.

Definitions: Current source density, inverse solution, signal to noise ratio, sinusoids, cross spectra

CHAPTER 1

Introduction
to LORETA

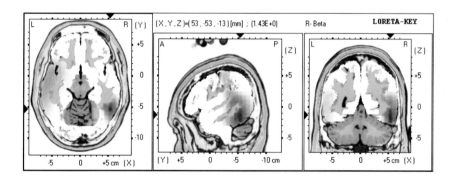

CHAPTER 1

Introduction to LORETA

Neuronal mechanisms and behavior continue to drive both the neuroscience and psychology fields. It has long been known that the brain is the central core of all human functions, be it cognitive, emotional, social, interpersonal, and intrapersonal. Of course, studying these specific functions and their respective neural assemblies presents a difficult challenge for scientists. Fortuitously, few innovators have combined the worlds of physics, mathematics, psychology, and biological sciences to facilitate significant advancements in the study of the brain. The developments in positron emission tomography (PET), magnetic resonance imaging (MRI), and functional magnetic resonance imaging (fMRI) techniques have exponentially increased our understanding of brain-behavior relationships. However, the specific mechanism of the electroencephalogram (EEG) has been somewhat restricted to surface evaluations and event-related potentials research, largely due to the nature of the inverse problem and the lack of a unique inverse solution.

The reliable localization of EEG sources within the brain presents complex problem involving propagation of electromagnetic waves and the measurement of the signals that can be accurately differentiated and localized to a specific brain region

(Hämäläinen, 1984; Lehmann, Michel, Pal, & Pascual-Marqui, 1994; Pascual-Marqui & Biscay-Lirio, 1993; Pascual-Marqui, Gonzalez-Andino, Valdes-Sosa, & Biscay-Lirio, 1988; Pascual-Marqui, Michel, & Lehmann, 1995; Pascual-Marqui, Valdes-Sosa, & Alvarez-Amador, 1988). The sources of the scalp EEG may be considered magnetic dipoles or distributed current sources for which the inverse problem must be solved (Lopes da Silva, 2004). Thus, source localization of the EEG has been an active research area in recent decades. Dr. Roberto Pascual-Marqui is the developer of the LORETA family. He is a successful researcher at the Key Institute for Brain-Mind Research at the University Hospital of Psychiatry in Zurich (the web address to obtain additional information and download the LORETA software program is http://www.uzh.ch/keyinst/loreta.htm).

Low-resolution electromagnetic tomography (LORETA - Key) is a collection of independent modules run in specific sequence in order to transform the raw EEG signal into LORETA images. It is one of the most extensively used algorithms for addressing the inverse solution for source localization of the EEG produced on the scalp. The EEG potentials on the scalp are measured in a linear fashion with respect to source amplitudes. In short, LORETA utilizes a fixed (finite) element method (FEM) to solve the Poisson equation that uses geometric information known about the layers of the brain, skull, and scalp as well as their conductivities (Sanei, 2007).

LORETA and the standardized version (sLORETA) are reliable inverse solutions for estimating cortical electrical current density originating from scalp electrodes that utilize optimal smoothing to estimate a direct 3D solution for the electrical activity distribution. This method computes distributed electrical activity within the cerebral volume, which is discretized and mapped onto a dense grid array containing sources of electrical activity at each point in the 3D grid with a low error solution for source generators.

LORETA generates statistical maps, models distribution currents of brain activity (Holmes, Brown, & Tucker, 2004; Lehmann et al., 2001; Lehmann et al., 2005; Lehmann,

Faber, Gianotti, Kochi, & Pascual-Marqui, 2006; Pascual-Marqui, Esslen, Kochi, & Lehmann, 2002; Pascual-Marqui et al., 1999), and utilizes realistic electrode coordinates (Towle et al., 1993) for a three-concentric-shell spherical head model co-registered on a standardized MRI atlas (Talairach, 1988). These procedures provide accurate approximation of anatomical labeling within the neocortical volume, including the anterior cingulate, hippocampus, and amygdaloid complex (Cannon, Lubar, Thornton, Wilson, & Congedo, 2005; Coutin-Churchman & Moreno, 2008; Esslen, Pascual-Marqui, Hell, Kochi, & Lehmann, 2004; Lancaster et al., 2000). LORETA operates under the assumption that the spatial gradient of voltage will change gradually and as such, it selects maximally smooth distribution of source magnitudes. The physiological justification underlying this constraint is that activity in neurons in neighboring patches of cortex is correlated.

Importantly, it has been demonstrated that LORETA provides better temporal resolution than can be achieved with either PET or fMRI (Kim et al., 2009), while PET and MRI offer superior spatial resolution. The advantage of EEG LORETA is that EEG is a direct measure of neuronal activity and its potential uses increase exponentially with the added spatial localization of 5mm with sLORETA. The temporal resolution is not only important for studies using event related potentials (i.e., time-locked events), but it is also very important for investigating state changes proposed to be elicited by psychological constructs. For example, consider the state elicited by attachment, depression, or other psychological measure and the duration that it may take to achieve a state change from resting baseline. Our laboratory, the Clinical Neuroscience, self-regulation, and biological psychology laboratory at the University of Tennessee, is currently pursuing these important research areas. Ultimately, combining these methods may prove important for integrating the "what and where" of the brain in normal cognitive processes and psychopathology (Cannon, 2009; Cannon, Baldwin, & Lubar, 2008; Cannon, Congedo, Lubar, & Hutchens, 2009; Cannon et al., 2007).

LORETA is accessible as freeware for research purposes and is the only inverse solution that has been employed for real-time neurofeedback use (Congedo, Lubar, & Joffe, 2004). LORETA has been shown to estimate current density sources efficiently with 19 electrodes (Congedo, 2006; Congedo et al., 2004; Lubar, Congedo, & Askew, 2003; Sherlin et al., 2007) and as few as 16, with maximum error of 10mm (Cohen et al., 1990; Pascual-Marqui, 1999). Current density is mapped for 2,394 voxels of 7mm^3 dimension, covering the entire neocortex and producing a maximum error of 14mm (Pascual-Marqui, 1999). The standardized version (sLORETA) is also freely available for research purposes and utilizes the standardized MRI atlas from the Montreal Neurological Institute (MNI), which consists of 6,329 brain volume elements (voxels) of 5mm^3. The sLORETA version proposes that 3-D source localization methods cannot improve the localization error beyond the present result (sLORETA). LORETA and sLORETA are easy to use once the mechanics are learned. While this manuscript is designed to provide the basics of LORETA and its applications in clinical and research settings, it is by no means exhaustive. A concise manual describing the use and application of LORETA and providing information about the brain and potential clinical targets for LORETA methods are the primary incentives for writing this manuscript.

1.1: LORETA: Basic Assumptions

Scientists typically employ two general approaches to the source localization of EEG. Equivalent current dipole (ECD) is an approach, which assumes that a small number of focal sources generate the EEG signals (Miltner, Braun, Johnson, Simpson, & Ruchkin, 1994; Scherg, 1994; Scherg & Ebersole, 1994; Scherg, Ille, Bornfleth, & Berg, 2002). Linearly distributed approaches consider all possible source localizations simultaneously (Hamalainen & Ilmoniemi, 1994; Phillips, Rugg, & Fristont, 2002; Sarvas, 1987). Inverse methods that use the dipole source model consider the source localizations as discrete magnetic dipoles in fixed positions within a three-dimensional space in the brain. The current distributed source reconstruction method requires no knowledge of the number of sources (for an excellent review on these topics see (Sanei, 2007). In the most basic terms, the electrode potentials and the matrix of source amplitudes and locations in 3-D space are considered to be linearly related by LORETA based on the superposition principle (Sanei, 2007).

In revisiting basic physics, the superposition principle holds that at any instant, the resultant combination wave is the algebraic sum of all component waves. Thus, two or more solutions to a linear equation or set of linear equations can be added together such that their sum is also a solution. These assumptions are often cited as criticisms of LORETA; thus, knowing these and reading more about the linear transformations as applied to waveforms will benefit the user. The debate about the use of linear functions will undoubtedly continue; however, it is quite reasonable to put forth the notion that the brain and its enigmatic mechanisms operate using both linear and non-linear properties in addition to undiscovered mechanisms. There simply is not enough evidence to support that either approach is better at describing the complex system known as the brain. It is best to know and understand the limitations and assumptions under which one is operating to promote responsible use of the LORETA software, including rigorous scrutiny of the drawn conclusions.

In the last few decades, neuroscience research has increased at an exponential rate. Positron Emission Tomography (PET) is an indirect measure of local neuronal activity (Raichle, 1998). Increased neural activity increases regional cerebral glucose metabolism (rCGM) to brain regions involved in mental activities or cognitively demanding tasks (Shulman et al., 1997; Shulman et al., 1999; Shulman, Ollinger, Linenweber, Petersen, & Corbetta, 2001). An indirect measure of functional magnetic resonance imaging (fMRI) produces the blood oxygenated level dependent (BOLD) response. Despite the advantages of increased spatial resolution, limitations regarding the temporal resolution and ambiguity associated with the interpretation and reporting of results remain (Logothetis, Pauls, Augath, Trinath, & Oeltermann, 2001; Logothetis & Wandell, 2004). There is often a high degree of overlap in activation of brain regions during cognitive, memory, attentional, and affective tasks, which adds to the difficulty in interpreting fMRI results (Cabeza & Nyberg, 2000). PET and fMRI provide very good spatial resolution; however, the researcher determines the interpretation of the signal increase in localizing a measurable regional increase while the reader often questions the meaning of this increase. Is it metabolic firing, neuronal firing, or both that cause this increase? More importantly, what EEG frequency domains might be at work during these experimental tasks? LORETA might be able to answer these questions. Particularly, the temporal quality of EEG and LORETA permit longer exposure to stimuli and facilitate the study of the brain over longer periods under more complex stimulus presentations.

1.2: LORETA: Validation Studies

Independent laboratories have conducted extensive validation of LORETA, including the mathematical proofs (Sekihara, Sahani, & Nagarajan, 2005; Wagner, Fuchs, & Kastner, 2004). Currently, over 750 research articles with keywords LORETA or low-resolution electromagnetic tomography are listed in PubMed. Thus, there is no shortage of references for case studies and research publications. This method finds a particular solution addressing the non-unique EEG inverse problem by assuming similar activation of neighboring neuronal sources, followed by an appropriate standardization of the current density, producing images of electric neuronal activity without localization bias (Greenblatt, Gan, Harmatz, & Shader, 2005; Pascual-Marqui, 2002; Sekihara, Sahani, & Nagarajan, 2005).

LORETA (Pascual-Marqui, Michel, & Lehmann, 1994) has received considerable validation from studies that combined this method with more established localization methods, including fMRI (Mulert et al., 2004; Vitacco, Brandeis, Pascual-Marqui, & Martin, 2002), structural MRI (Worrell et al., 2000), PET (Oakes et al., 2004; Zumsteg, Wennberg, Treyer, Buck, & Wieser, 2005), and invasive implanted electrode recordings (Zumsteg, Andrade, & Wennberg, 2006). The results from these as well as other studies validate sLORETA as an improved version of the original LORETA method. It has also been demonstrated that LORETA can correctly localize deep structures, such as the anterior cingulate cortex (Pizzagalli, Oakes, & Davidson, 2003) and mesial temporal lobes (Zumsteg et al., 2006).

1.3: Basic Electroencephalogram Primer

Richard Caton first used electroencephalogram (EEG) in 1875 to record spontaneous electrical activity occurring in the brains of animals (Brazier, 1961). Hans Berger recorded the first human EEG in 1924 (Berger, 1929). EEG signals are direct signatures of neuronal activity that can be recorded in different formats from different locations on the scalp, inside the brain, and in between the brain and scalp. It has been proposed that the EEG recorded from the scalp is derived from excitatory (EPSP) and inhibitory (IPSP) post synaptic potentials, or that millisecond scale modulations of synaptic current sources at the surfaces of neocortical neurons generate rather large scale cortical and scalp potentials (Nunez, 2006). Further, EEG rhythms are proposed to correspond to the synchronized synaptic activity of large numbers of neurons across neural pathways (or networks) and can be thought of in terms of harmonics. The EEG at any given point is a complex summation of many frequencies that are additive or subtractive in nature. Differential patterns of waveforms may represent specific functionality. However, specific functions of EEG oscillatory activity still involve much uncertainty (Zschocke, 2000). The suggestion that synchronization of distributed neural networks functionally integrates differential brain structures (Bushara et al., 2003) is an important direction for further study. The EEG or electrical activity of the brain is measured in the form of waves with specific bands of frequencies measured in hertz (Hz), measuring typical amplitude ranges in microvolts (μV). Five major EEG frequency bands are differentiated by their ranges described as delta (0.5-3.5 Hz; 20-200 μV), theta (3.5-7.5 Hz; 20-100 μV), alpha (7.5-13 Hz; 20-60 μV), beta (13-30 Hz; 2-20 μV), and gamma (30-100 Hz, 0.01-1 μV) waves (D'Angiulli, Grunau, Maggi, & Herdman, 2006). Researchers utilize different variations of these frequency bands; however, the amplitudes on the scalp that these frequency domains exhibit range from 0.10 to 100 microvolts (μV). In addition, EEG activity can be quantified as power (i.e., magnitude squared, $μV^2$ units) within a frequency band graphed as a function of time.

Additionally, synchrony can be used to describe EEG patterns. During sleep, the EEG is dominated by increased (high-voltage) and slow (<3 Hz) electrical activity (synchronized) that can be expressed as a percentage increase in EEG activity, while during alert wakefulness, the EEG shows a pattern of decreased (low-voltage) and fast (>12 Hz) electrical activity (desynchronized) that can be expressed as a percentage decrease in EEG activity.

1.4: The Delta Frequency Domain (0.5 - 3.5 Hz)

In normal populations, the delta frequency is most notably associated with the onset of sleep (Lubin, Nute, Naitoh, & Martin, 1973). However, it is also suggested that delta activity plays a particular role in information encoding and retrieval as well as in overall intelligence (Knyazev, Savostyanov, & Levin, 2005; Kurova & Cheremushkin, 2007). Teylor (1989) examined the development of long-term potentiation in the hippocampus and in neocortex of the rat. He found that while maximal potentiation in hippocampal synapses occurred with stimulation in the gamma (100-400 Hz) frequency band, bursts in both delta (2 Hz) and gamma (100 Hz) bands resulted in maximal long term-potentiation in the neocortex (Teyler, 1989). In a recent review, Steriade focused on evidence that activity of neocortical neurons during slow-wave sleep is associated with neuronal plasticity and may play a role in consolidating memory traces acquired during the waking state (Steriade, 2004). Klimesch, Hanslmayr, Sauseng, Gruber, Brozinsky, Kroll and colleagues (2006) identified a role of delta frequency activity in a two stage encoding process occurring between repeated learning trials. Based on LORETA source localization, the authors concluded that two different stages could characterize episodic encoding. Traces are first processed at parietal sites at approximately 300 ms. Then, further processing takes place in regions of the medial temporal lobe at approximately 500 ms. Only the first stage is associated with theta, whereas the second is characterized by a slow wave with a frequency of approximately 2.5 Hz (Klimesch et al., 2006).

Memory impairment is the most common difficulty reported by survivors of traumatic brain injury (TBI). Converging evidence suggests that this complaint is associated with alterations in functional cerebral activity (Christodoulou et al., 2001). The frontal lobes, especially the left hemisphere, are implicated in various mnemonic, language, and auditory processes. Typically, studies associate theta frequency, a prominent feature in the hippocampal formation, with memory processes (Machulda et al., 2003). However, higher cognitive functioning is reported to involve slow synchronization of delta or theta frequency range over longer distances (Lubar, 1997), while faster frequency bands are reported to involve local neuronal populations (Chow & Kopell, 2000; Jones, Pinto, Kaper, & Kopell, 2000; Kopell, Ermentrout, Whittington, & Traub, 2000; White, Banks, Pearce, & Kopell, 2000).

Delta activity is reportedly involved in the P3b of the P300 and is active in parietal P300 during rare stimuli presentation tasks (Kolev, Demiralp, Yordanova, Ademoglu, & Isoglu-Alkac, 1997; Yordanova & Kolev, 1997). Often, high amplitude, synchronized delta activity is indicative of TBI or other insult (e.g., stroke, minimal cognitive state). The plastic neural functioning component of the delta frequency domains is of considerable interest as it pertains to compensatory brain activation patterns, in individuals with TBI. Delta may prove to play an important role in communication and language functions between subcortical regions, limbic system and cortex (Akila, Muller, Kaukiainen, & Sainio, 2006; Krause et al., 2006; Muller & Knight, 2006; Werkle-Bergner, Muller, Li, & Lindenberger, 2006).

Recent data indicate that the sources of delta activity in Alzheimer's disease and mild cognitive impairment correlate negatively with frontal white matter volumes (Babiloni, et al., 2006), stressing the importance of delta activity in functional connectivity within the brain and possible detection of such measures as diagnostic indicators. Since delta is often thought of as specific to sleep, cortical reorganization during the sleep cycle perhaps reflects a marked loss of coherence within the hippocampus during sleep, which suggests that the lower frequencies of delta and theta operate more independently in sleep cycles (Brazier, 1968). Slower frequencies are reportedly present in the limbic system and limbic structures, as the amygdala and hippocampus tend to develop their own spindling patterns independent of the cortex (Brazier, 1968).

Arousal is associated with widespread cortical and hippocampal desynchronization or decreased phase synchrony globally. Evoked potentials of sensory stimulation are large and widespread over the cortex, which may imply that the role of arousal and the salience of a stimulus relate to its significance not necessarily to its intensity. Thus, we might consider that the behavioral reaction (cortical event), which involves receiving, coding, classifying, and perceiving (interpreting) the stimulus, occurs during stimulus presentation. Much work needs to be done to clarify this notion. However, it might be considered that delta plays an important part in this type of function due to its prominence in the limbic system (Smythies, 1966) and the associated connections from the reticular formation. The delta frequency has not been thought of as important to cognitive processes or a target of neuromodulation techniques; however, as the mysteries associated with this frequency domain are unraveled, it may be that delta plays an important role in cognitive functioning as well as emotion and regulatory processes with cross-frequency co-modulation properties.

1.5: The Theta Frequency Domain (3.5 - 7.5 Hz)

The theta frequency is most notably associated with memory processes. It also plays a role in information encoding and retrieval as well as executive attention (Cannon, Congedo, Lubar, & Hutchens, 2009; Cannon et al., 2007). Theta is also a predominant frequency associated with the cingulate gyrus in both anterior and posterior regions, with hippocampal theta activity being the primary contributor to this phenomenon (Borst, Leung, & MacFabe, 1987; Leung & Borst, 1987). Moreover, in combination with the gamma frequency, theta seems to play an intricate role in reward, motivation, and cognitive processing (Klimesch, 1999; Klimesch et al., 2006; Klimesch, Schack, & Sauseng, 2005; Knyazev et al., 2005; Lehmann, Henggeler, Koukkou, & Michel, 1993), in addition to the possible governance of cognitive processes (Basar, Basar-Eroglu, Karakas, & Schurmann, 1999, 2001) as well as visual encoding and retrieval processes (Fink & Neubauer, 2006; Schmid, Tirsch, & Scherb, 2002; Thatcher, North, & Biver, 2008).

Previous findings suggest that oscillations within the theta frequency band (~4 - 8 Hz) (Klimesch, Doppelmayr, Schimke, & Ripper, 1997; Klimesch, Doppelmayr, Schwaiger, Auinger, & Winkler, 1999) in a hippocampal-cortical loop system (Burgess & Gruzelier, 1997; Fell et al., 2003; Klimesch, 1996) reflect the encoding of episodic (short term) and working memory processes. During encoding, the increase in theta is significantly larger for items that can later be remembered (Klimesch, 1996; Klimesch et al., 2001). Theta amplitude also increases with increasing memory load during a memory retention interval, reflecting a specific role of theta in maintenance of the memory trace. Moreover, theta synchronization is maximal during retrieval in which the amplitude of theta synchronization predicts retrieval success (Fingelkurts, Krause, & Sams, 2002; Jensen & Tesche, 2002;

Klimesch, 1999). Thus, an explicit role of theta has been identified in encoding, retention, and retrieval of a memory trace (Klimesch, 2000). Lower theta amplitude at rest and higher amplitude during learning performance (reflecting a large increase in theta power during task) has been demonstrated to predict good memory performance (Klimesch, 1999; Klimesch, Doppelmayr, Pachinger, & Ripper, 1997).

Corticocortical and thalamocortical neural networks generate mainly the alpha rhythm (~8-12 Hz) (Klimesch, Doppelmayr, Schimke, et al., 1997; Klimesch, Schimke, & Schwaiger, 1994; Steriade, Gloor, Llinas, de Silva, & Mesulam, 1990). Research suggests distinct roles of lower (~8-10 Hz) and upper (~10-12 Hz) alpha band activity in cognition and attention. The lower band relates primarily to response readiness and attentional demands (Klimesch et al., 1992), and it is proposed to play only an indirect role in memory. By contrast, oscillations in the upper alpha band have been consistently observed during (semantic) long-term memory processes (Klimesch, Doppelmayr, Russegger, & Pachinger, 1996; Klimesch, Doppelmayr, Russegger, Pachinger, & Schwaiger, 1998; Klimesch et al., 1994). In contrast to the theta band, higher alpha amplitude at rest and lower alpha amplitude during task performance (reflecting a large alpha suppression during task) correlate with efficient memory performance in healthy adult subjects (Klimesch, 1999; Klimesch, Doppelmayr, Pachinger, et al., 1997; Stipacek, Grabner, Neuper, Fink, & Neubauer, 2003; Vogt, Klimesch, & Doppelmayr, 1998).

This comodulation or cross-frequency coupling activity may be more specific to functional encoding of information from regions involved in spatial orientation. It may also be attributed to the involvement of posterior regions in the evaluation of visual and sensory information and encoding into memory, since theta oscillations (Klimesch, Doppelmayr, Schimke, et al., 1997; Klimesch et al., 1999) within a thalamo-hippocampal-cortical system seem to reflect the encoding of episodic (short term) and working memory processes (Burgess & Gruzelier, 1997; Fell et al., 2003; Klimesch, 1996). Encoding significantly increases theta for items that can be remembered later (Klimesch, 1996; Klimesch et al., 2001). Delta and theta power have been shown to increase in frontal regions during working memory tasks (Aguirre-Perez, Otero-Ojeda, Pliego-Rivero, & Ferreira-Martinez, 2007). Similarly, and of particular emphasis, short term memory tasks increase gamma power in frontal and parietal regions with directionality shown as frontal to parietal, suggesting that frontal areas would influence memory retention in parietal regions (Babiloni et al., 2004).

Left temporal increase in theta power has been shown during lexical retrieval tasks (Bastiaansen, van der Linden, Ter Keurs, Dijkstra, & Hagoort, 2005). The delta frequency has been posited to be instrumental in attention to internal states during mental tasks (Harmony et al., 1996); similarly, delta, theta and alpha 2 activity have been shown to be involved in internal speech, rehearsal of verbal working memory in left temporal-parietal regions, and dorsolateral prefrontal regions (Harmony et al., 1999). Klimesch et al. (2003) utilized repetitive transcranial magnetic stimulation (rTMS) to induce increased upper alpha activity during a reference interval preceding the performance of a working memory task. Their findings indicated that only rTMS in the upper alpha frequency band (defined as a frequency of 1 Hz above peak individual alpha frequency, termed IAF) lead to a significant improvement in working memory performance when compared with control conditions. Klimesch and colleagues applied rapid rate repetitive transcranial magnetic stimulation (rTMS) immediately preceding a mental rotation task. Stimulation was delivered at three different frequencies to fronto-central and right parietal sites identified in previous studies as active during a mental rotation task. Sham stimulation was also delivered to the parietal site. They found that rTMS delivered in the upper alpha frequency range to either the fronto-central or right parietal site resulted in improved cognitive performance during task while neither sham stimulation nor stimulation at lower alpha and mid-beta frequencies had significant effect on task accuracy (Klimesch, Sauseng, & Gerloff, 2003).

Kohler and colleagues investigated the effect of rTMS in the upper theta (7 Hz) frequency range on list learning efficiency. Utilizing two stage methodology, they first used fMRI to localize activation to the left inferior prefrontal cortex (LIPFC) related to semantic encoding in 12 subjects. Consequently, they administered rTMS to the same subjects during performance of the semantic encoding task, targeting for stimulation the areas specific to each subject identified by fMRI as active during semantic list learning. They reported that words encoded under LIPFC stimulation were subsequently recognized with higher accuracy compared to words encoded under stimulation at two control sites. They attributed their findings to the triggering of more extensive processing of stimulated items as well as to the physiological processes of facilitation (Kohler, Paus, Buckner, & Milner, 2004). The theta frequency has received a great deal of attention from researchers in the recent past due in part to its prominence in hippocampal and cingulate regions. In a recent work, we attempted to train individuals to increase theta activity in the dorsal anterior cingulate gyrus. Participants were able to increase the amplitude of theta; however, as the amplitude increased, so did episodes of tear production. This began to interfere with the recording procedures; therefore, we adjusted the protocol to low-beta power, improving the results. Interestingly, participants did not report emotional distress (e.g., sadness, depression) only increased tear production. Our future research efforts will seek to expand upon this phenomenon.

1.6: The Alpha Frequency Domain (7.5 - 12.0 Hz)

The alpha frequency is proposed to be generated in thalamic regions and involved in processes of retrieval, scanning, and accessing information from declarative memory stores (Klimesch, 1997). Alpha activity is thought to be involved in all variants of attention, including alerting, orienting and sustaining attention, as well as visual processing and cognitive preparedness (Angelakis, Lubar, & Stathopoulou, 2004; Angelakis, Lubar, Stathopoulou, & Kounios, 2004; Cannon et al., 2009; Cannon et al., 2007). Additionally, alpha has been shown to play a role in evaluation of self and mental state decoding as well as working memory (Cannon, Lubar, & Baldwin, 2008; Sabbagh & Flynn, 2006). The theta frequency has also been shown to correlate with working memory subtests of the Wechsler Adult Intelligence Scale (Polunina & Davydov, 2006). Klimesch et al. (1997) demonstrated that theta and desynchronization in the upper alpha frequency band correlate with semantic memory processes. It is unclear how specific frequencies interact with specific regions to facilitate memory; however, as mentioned earlier, synchronization and desynchronization of local and long distance neuronal populations may be the key to this mechanism (Klimesch, 1997; Klimesch, Doppelmayr, Pachinger, et al., 1997; Klimesch, Doppelmayr, Schimke, et al., 1997).

Changes in the alpha rhythm may represent various important cognitive functions, including encoding, retrieval, and information processing (Doppelmayr, Klimesch, Hodlmoser, Sauseng, & Gruber, 2005; Doppelmayr, Klimesch, Sauseng, et al., 2005; Gruber, Klimesch, Sauseng, & Doppelmayr, 2005; Sauseng, Klimesch, Doppelmayr, et al., 2005; Sauseng et al., 2006; Sauseng, Klimesch, Schabus, & Doppelmayr, 2005; Sauseng, Klimesch, Stadler, et al., 2005). Moreover, selective bands within the alpha frequency also seem to play a particular role in attention and working memory, with the lower alpha band (8 - 10 Hz) being associated with attention and the higher alpha band (10 - 12 Hz) with working memory processes (Sauseng, Klimesch, Doppelmayr, et al., 2005). Alpha band power was also detected as having frontal (anterior cingulate) and limbic variants that are, like posterior alpha rhythms, not susceptible to suppression by anxiolytics (Connemann et al., 2005). Interestingly, the hallmark signature of EEG changes due to dementia of the Alzheimer's type are a general slowing and decrease in alpha activity and an increase in theta activity. Cognitive decline has been shown to be associated with changes in higher frequency domains in occipital and temporal regions, and such changes have been shown to correlate with disease severity (Jeong, 2004). Posterial commissural fibers within the corpus callosum have shown the strongest correlation with the alpha frequency, such that the

Isthmus and Tapetum in the superior occipital cortex show the highest positive association with the alpha frequency. Data suggests that cortico-thalamocortical cycles may modulate the alpha frequency domain while white matter architecture is associated more with the alpha frequency domain than with neocortical region or grey matter (Valdes-Hernandez et al., 2010). Compared to normal controls, recent data for recovering substance abusers demonstrated an increase in alpha activity in right limbic and orbital frontal regions during the evaluation of self (Cannon, Baldwin, & Lubar, 2008). This finding and findings of other studies on depression (Paquette, Beauregard, & Beaulieu-Prevost, 2009), anxiety (Isotani et al., 2001; Milad & Rauch, 2007), and experiences that created intense anger (Cannon, Lubar, Thornton, Wilson, & Congedo, 2005) emphasize the potential role of higher EEG frequency domains of the limbic system in homeostatic and emotional anomalies (limbic irritability) involved in these particular syndromes. Further research should expand on this notion.

1.7: The Beta Frequency Domain (13 - 32 Hz)

Beta activity is proposed to be involved in affect, cognition and attention, as well as in executive functions and psychopathology (Clarke et al., 2007; Ray & Cole, 1985; Spironelli, Penolazzi, & Angrilli, 2008). Studies report an increase in local coherence of the beta 2 range (beta 1 = 14 -18 Hz, beta 2 = 18 – 21 Hz, beta 3 = 21 – 24 Hz, beta 4 = 24 – 28 Hz, beta 5 = 28 – 32 Hz) in the left frontal regions extending to the central area and of the beta 3 band mainly in the right frontal regions extending to central and anterior-medial temporal areas during imagery and language thought processes (Petsche, Lacroix, Lindner, Rappelsberger, & Schmidt-Henrich, 1992). Although it is not yet possible to assign a specific functional role to each frequency, the presence of beta and gamma oscillations is thought to represent an activated state of the underlying neuronal network.

These beta and gamma brain rhythms involve γ-aminobutyric acid type A (GABA$_A$)

receptor activity, yet researchers propose that it is difficult to assign any specific function to these higher frequency domains due to the changes in the alpha rhythm and the possibility that beta and gamma oscillations accompany alpha increases (Lansbergen, Arns, van Dongen-Boomsma, Spronk, & Buitelaar, 2010). Historically, it has been proposed that beta activity indicates a stimulated and actively engaged state; however, this has yet to be confirmed. Moreover, in our work on LORETA neurofeedback, we have found cross-frequency correlations that occur after training one specific frequency range (e.g., 14 - 18 Hz). Although the training itself produced significant changes in working memory and processing speed scores, we cannot rule out the possibility of interdependency between EEG frequency domains. For example, in our work on ADHD and Autism, we may train alpha specifically at a site. Upon monitoring changes throughout the brain and in specific regions of interest, we would discover correlations (positive or negative) between EEG frequencies.

Another example of this effect concerns up-training alpha. As alpha increases in amplitude, some frequencies show similar effects (delta, SMR, low-beta and beta-2) while other frequencies show inverse effects (beta 3 and theta). This simply raises questions that individuals who utilize the methods in this text need to consider. What do these correlations indicate? If these frequencies are correlated, interdependent phenomena, then are the methods that we have been using to analyze them correct? Beta is present when an individual is awake and alert, and this effect has been noted across species. As such, the EEG as well as its functions and interdependencies are certainly important areas for further study.

1.8: Artifacts and LORETA

Artifacts are an extremely important consideration for both quantitative EEG and LORETA. Paradoxically, there is an inherent minimization of intra-cranial noise by restricting the use to 19 channels such that the higher the number of electrodes increases the smoothness required by LORETA to localize the source (Congedo, Lotte, & Lecuyer, 2006; Congedo et al., 2004). This is demonstrated by cross-validation procedures, which emphasize that the production of extra-cranial artifacts poses a serious problem (Anderer, Saletu, Semlitsch, & Pascual-Marqui, 2003; Pascual-Marqui, 2002; Pascual-Marqui et al., 2002; Pascual-Marqui & Lehmann, 1993b; Pascual-Marqui, 1999). Since these artifacts are not constant over time, their effect on the validity of the current density estimation is great in both absolute and relative terms (Congedo, 2003). Therefore, the reference-independence property of LORETA is more than a simple technical issue because an active electrode records the potential difference between the active electrode and the location of the reference electrode (preferably, where the contribution of EEG to the signal is minimal). Different reference locations produce different effects on the EEG, including spectral power, coherence, and phase measurements (Essl & Rappelsberger, 1998; Fein, Raz, Brown, & Merrin, 1988; Nunez et al., 1997; Nunez, 2006; Pascual-Marqui & Lehmann, 1993a; Rappelsberger, 1989). These confounds are minimal in the LORETA program, given that the current density estimation is the same for any choice of common cranial reference (Pascual-Marqui et al., 1999; Pascual-Marqui, 1999). The results across laboratories may be more consistent because of this property. It is important that the fields of both EEG and neurofeedback give the utmost attention to the consistency of procedures.

Artifacts are the most formidable constant factors in EEG procedures. However, waveforms associated with artifact production are not constant since the EEG is sensitive to microvolt levels and electrical properties of events occurring outside of the skull. Eye-movements, eyelids, and forehead muscles, which can produce alterations in respective electrodes thereby producing disturbances in ambient electrical fields, also produce frontal artifacts. This is also true for tongue and jaw movements or tension in regions associated with temporal and parietal electrodes. Electrocardiogram (ECG), sweating, medical equipment, electrode shorting or popping, and disturbances between electrode pairs are other potential artifacts that may affect the EEG.

Many artifacts are recognized because of their characteristic appearance in the EEG record and their respective effects on the true EEG. Muscle activity and eye-movements maintain biphasic properties, such that high microvolt levels will diminish the true EEG signal. Similarly, artifacts show great variation, such that they may be single episodes or recurrent waves while others may be prolonged disturbances, such as sweating. The jaws typically show spiked, fast activity when clinched. However, tongue movements can produce slower, combination waves, which can contaminate parietal and central leads often used as a reference. Sweating also produces slow, prolonged waves that may resemble delta activity or slow cortical potentials. Eye movements, on the other hand, produce high amplitude waves, typically within the 1 - 4 Hz band, and these artifacts may be associated with blinking, eye-movement, body movement, and the electrical charge of the eye itself (Durka, Klekowicz, Blinowska, Szelenberger, & Niemcewicz, 2003; Elbert, Lutzenberger, Rockstroh, & Birbaumer, 1985; Fortgens & De Bruin, 1983; Joyce, Gorodnitsky, & Kutas, 2004; Koskinen & Vartiainen, 2009; W. Nakamura, et al., 2006; Shigemura, Nishimura, Tsubai, & Yokoi, 2004; Wallstrom, Kass, Miller, Cohn, & Fox, 2004). ECG produces small, recurrent spikes that are more visible in monopolar montages.

When dealing with artifacts in the EEG, several methods are utilized to correct or average out problematic elements, such as independent component analysis (ICA) or blind source separation (BSS). Although this section will not provide a comprehensive review of artifact detection and removal from the EEG stream since this has been done in other works (Thornton, 1995), it will provide examples of artifacts and methods to determine the influence of mentioned elements on the localization of sources in LORETA. In other words, it will identify artifacts associated with regions on the scalp and address the ways in which these artifacts may produce errors in localization. The LORETA Key package clearly states that the operator is responsible for the quality of the EEG to be analyzed since the software does not possess the ability to determine artifact from EEG, it simply performs the algorithm on the provided data; thus, if "garbage goes in, garbage will come out."

When considering artifacts associated with regional activations, for example regions in the prefrontal cortex increasing relative to attention or working memory processes, we find that it is important to understand features associated with artifacts and to remove their influence or in many cases, simply acknowledge their existence and adjust hypothetical notions accordingly. The delta frequency is a very good example. Artifacts produced by the large muscles of the neck and jaw may be confused with genuine delta frequency, as both ocular movements and blinking produce similar effects. Figure 1 illustrates an example of eye-blinks and their effects throughout the EEG recording.

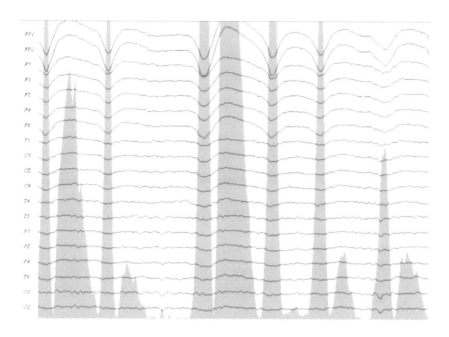

Figure 1: EEG recording with eye-blinks and eye-movement. The ordinate shows the electrode, the gray is the power spectrum. The artifacts occur in the delta frequency (between 1.0 and 3.5 with the peak at 3.0 Hz) and bleed into nearly all other electrodes.

This is a 19-channel, linked ear and ground reference recording that includes only ocular movements and blinks. This segment is 6 seconds in length. The amplitude of these artifacts is > 150 μV. Figure 2 below shows the LORETA results for this segment of ocular artifacts, indicating that delta deserves special consideration in the preparation of EEG files to be entered into LORETA analysis. Figures 1, 2, 3, and 4 show artifacts in the EEG stream and their effects on the LORETA calculations. Figure 3 illustrates an example of EMG artifact. The image shows artifacts recorded at temporal leads in the higher frequency domains, also showing transient slow artifacts present in frontal leads. Figure 5 shows an example of rather clean EEG during an eyes-closed recording.

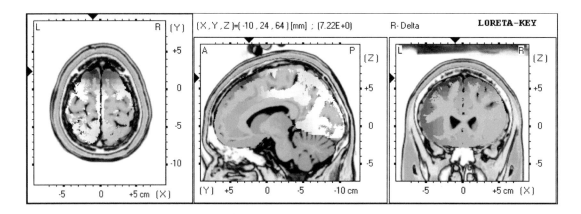

Figure 2: LORETA map of the 6-second segment of ocular artifact. The artifacts are mapped onto the frontal cortex as delta activity, extending into parietal and occipital regions. Additionally, the artifact includes central locations that are often used as an average reference (e.g., FZ, CZ, and PZ). It should also be noted that other frequency domains follow a similar pattern. Thus, the frontal leads require special attention concerning ocular movements and blinks.

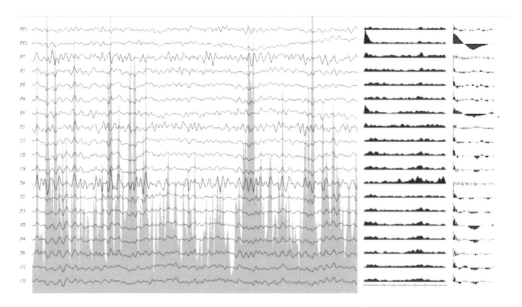

Figure 3: EMG artifact in 6-second section of EEG. The artifacts include F7, T3, and T4 in addition to eye movements in Fp2 and slight effects in Fp1. The artifacts appear to engage numerous parietal and occipital channels and thus the power spectrum is increased and the autocorrelation between waveforms (blue) is lessened. EMG and EOG tend to operate in a biphasic manner (an initial increase of the effect variable (delta) followed by a decrease at higher concentrations) and do not present sinusoidal form, as shown in Figure 5 below.

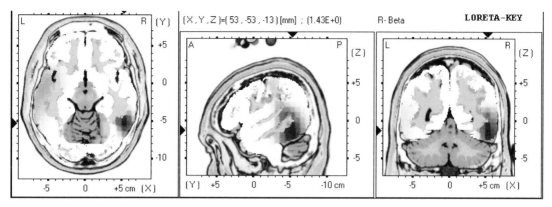

Figure 4: LORETA maps of EMG artifact shown in Figure 3. The LORETA estimation shows increased beta activity in the right temporal lobe, which obviously cannot be concluded due to artifact contamination mapped at T4.

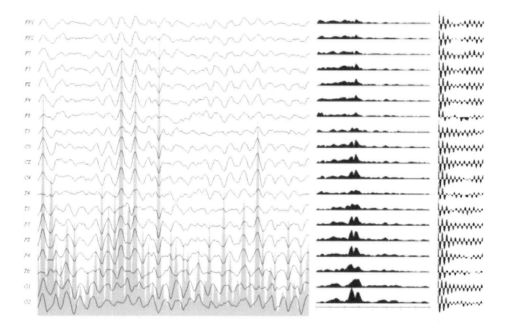

Figure 5: Two-second epoch of eyes-closed recording with minimal disturbances at F8, T4, and T6.

Importantly, many studies focus on memory and other functions associated with the temporal lobes. As such, these regions are very important for maintaining artifact free data, since the frontal and temporal regions may also contain artifacts that will be presented as activity in the beta or gamma frequency band. These artifacts can be anywhere between the 14 - 20 Hz range up to 35 - 55 Hz range. It is proposed that monitoring and removal of electromyography (EMG) spikes in the range of 10 - 15 microvolts indicates appreciable detection and removal criteria (Johnson, Wright, & Segall, 1979). This emphasizes the importance of the recording procedure, minimizing artifact production and the need for training and practice in recognizing artifacts.

1.9: Summary

LORETA is a valid and accurate method for localization of the EEG produced on the scalp. It is a fixed element method that assumes a linear relationship between potential sources of EEG activity. LORETA finds a direct solution for the electric activity distribution with only minimal sacrifice in spatial localization. It provides a much more accurate temporal resolution and offers the potential to investigate cognitive, affective, and perceptual processes that may not be susceptible to investigation by other neuroimaging techniques. It may be argued that spatial resolution is an inherent obstacle to using inverse solutions such as LORETA; however, research has proposed that fMRI spatial resolution in certain experimental conditions is maximized at 0.8 - 1.2 cm in the somatosensory cortex (Ozcan, Baumgartner, Vucurevic, Stoeter, & Treede, 2005). On the other hand, LORETA and localization of the EEG may be 1cm or less, as proposed by Nunez (Nunez, 1981). Furthermore, sLORETA provides mechanisms to extrapolate current source density (CSD) levels from ROI consisting of 5mm^3 in order to provide systematic evaluation of network functionality.

Artifacts are an important consideration for the user of LORETA; therefore, special attention needs to be given to frontal and temporal leads before analyzing EEG data in LORETA. Similarly, as the user engages in clinical use of LORETA, an increased knowledge base of functional neuroanatomy is required. This should include advanced training in neurophysiology, neuroanatomy, as well as neuroendocrine and metabolic processes.

LORETA is also an exceptional method for exploring functional connectivity within the cerebral volume and describing correlations between brain regions in terms of EEG frequency domains. LORETA along with other neuroimaging techniques provides an opportunity to further our knowledge of the brain and the intricacies of this most complex of complex systems. The EEG still contains many uncertainties and in many ways, we do not understand the basic mechanisms and characteristics of these phenomena. Further studies need to address the possibility that the EEG frequencies are interdependent; therefore, it is unlikely that any random or spontaneous noise is occurring, including artifacts. In short, all activity seen on the EEG record may be relative to experimental stimuli and have a significant meaning when analyzed in such a way as to accommodate violations of independence. This discipline still has to examine many unanswered questions.

CHAPTER 2

LORETA Interface and Modules

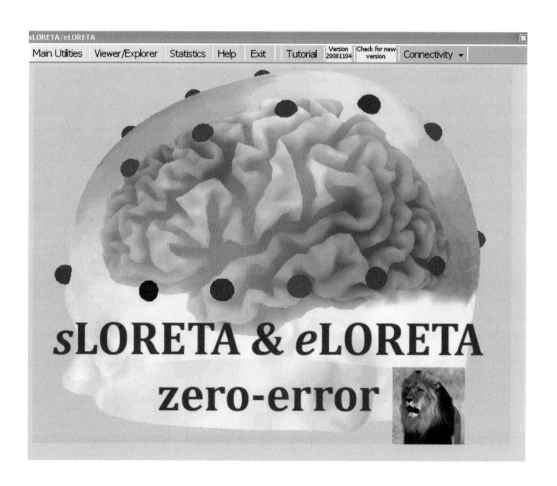

CHAPTER 2

LORETA Interface and Modules

In the following sections, I will describe and provide specific examples using each of the modules within the LORETA Key package and sLORETA, from download and installation to statistical comparisons. In short, I will cover electrode coordinates, transformation matrix, cross-spectral matrices, transforming the EEG/CRS files to LORETA images, and functional uses of this data. It is my desire to facilitate an increased use of EEG LORETA in both clinical and research settings in order to develop interest in using this or other types of technology to demonstrate evidence based treatment outcomes. Once downloaded, the LORETA program installs all necessary components in the C:/ Programs directory. All Modules in the program folder are accessible from the LORETA main screen shown in Figure 6. LORETA also installs file folders for each module in the C://Programfiles/LORETA/directory - all modules can be run from this location as well as the main screen. Help files are also available for each of these modules in the file folders or from the main screen.

In this chapter, I demonstrate the utilization of many different aspects of EEG in various components within LORETA. For ease of use and readability, this text does not discuss these methods in detail. Instead, it provides a guide for practical and clinical use.

Discussion of the mathematics and physics involved in estimations, such as cross-spectra, transformation matrices, and current source density estimations, are beyond the scope of this text. The reader is encouraged to examine (Nunez, 2006) and other such texts for explication on the methods discussed. Figure 6 shows the main screen of the LORETA program. On the left are all modules included in the program. These can be expanded and then the appropriate module can be selected.

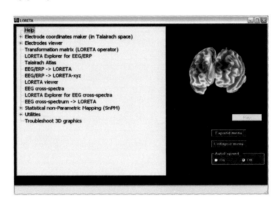

Figure 6: LORETA main screen. Access to all modules is provided in this interface.

Figure 7 shows the contents of the LORETA folder. All modules shown in the main screen can also be accessed from each of the folders. A note: The folder shown in this Figure 7 is associated with software installed from www.novatecheeg.com and as such, it contains additional components that will not be present in the stand-alone LORETA package (e.g., Mhyt, EUREKA! and associated files).

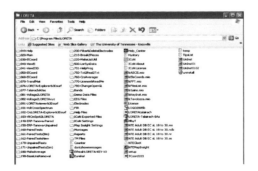

Figure 7: LORETA program folder and modules included. The modules for LORETA have a unique folder. The extra components in this folder (Eureka!, Mhyt, are from installation of software by www. novatecheeg.com).

2.1: Electrodes

The LORETA electrode maker creates a file with the electrode coordinates for the corresponding EEG files to be used in the analysis. For all modules henceforth, it is necessary to specify the number of electrodes, the number of time frames in each EEG file, and the sampling rate. Figure 8 shows the electrode coordinate maker in LORETA. In the image, active electrodes are selected according to the international 10/20 system (Jasper, 1958). Creating the electrode coordinates file is a necessary step for all subsequent modules. The electrode order in the list must match the electrode order (montage) according to the device that collected the EEG data. Once selected, the electrode is shown in red on the map while unselected electrodes remain blue. After selecting all electrodes, this file can be saved by clicking the save tab in the menu bar and named for further use.

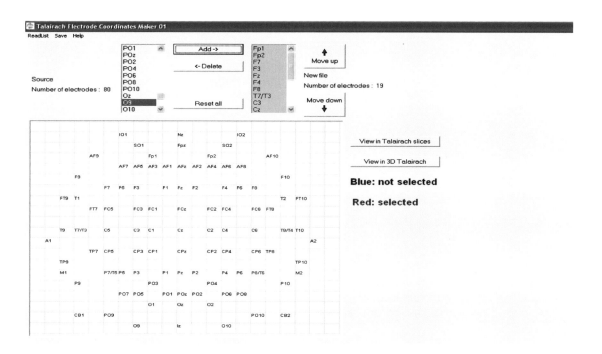

Figure 8: Electrode coordinates (19 channels) maker interface in LORETA. The selected electrodes are red, while unselected electrodes remain blue. The user can save the file by clicking the save option in the menu bar after naming the file.

2.2: Cross-Spectra

The LORETA cross-spectra module contains its own help file. The cross spectra module operates in two capacities. It can compute the cross spectra for individual EEG files or for a group of EEG files. The EEG cross spectra is computed using a parametric model for multi-channel EEG data (Pascual-Marqui, Valdes-Sosa, et al., 1988). In the most basic sense, the EEG is a collection of time series comprised of any number of time instants or discrete frequency ranges. EEG segments are referred to as epochs that typically range from 2 to 8 seconds, depending on the equipment and data collection parameters. In order to compute the cross-spectra, the user must include the number of electrodes, the number of time frames in each EEG file, and the sampling rate. The various frequency range options can also be entered in the settings. These settings contain typical frequencies; although, the user may enter discrete frequency ranges. An option is available to normalize the EEG, which implies that the EEG is normalized to total global field power (GFP) prior to the computation of the spectra. In short, the GFP is the sum of squared electric potentials over all electrodes and time frames. Figure 9 (next page) shows the EEG cross spectra viewer in the LORETA explorer window accessed from the main screen with the aforementioned functions in tab form.

Figure 10 (on page 36) shows the EEG/ERP LORETA explorer. (To use this module, the electrode file and transformation matrix (TM) (see below) must be completed first.) The image shows the EEG waveforms, electrodes, the global field power (GFP), and local GFP. One opens the EEG by selecting the file from the particular folder in which the EEG collection device stored it. To view the scalp map, the user must also open the electrode coordinates and TM files created earlier. The user then selects reference electrode, filter and band pass settings. The requested EEG/ERP files are text (txt.) files with no headers or footers. These text files must have a number of rows equal to the number of time frames or discrete time samples. Similarly the number of columns should equal the number of electrodes (columns = electrodes/ rows = time samples). Figure 11 (next page) shows the LORETA cross-spectra viewer. This module permits the user to view the square root of cross spectra and generators of EEG frequency components.

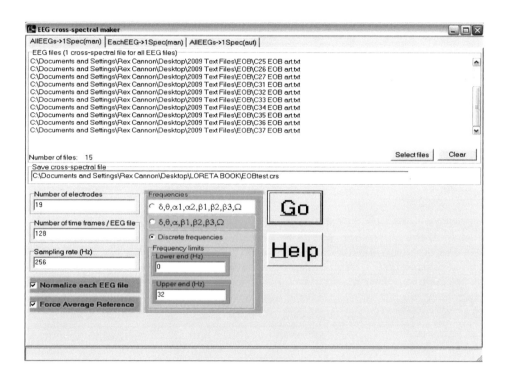

Figure 9: EEG cross spectra maker module. The selected EEG text files are in the top window. Below this window, the user clicks on the tab to define where the output file will be stored. Next, the number of electrodes, time frames, and sampling rate are entered in the form fields, and options are selected to normalize the EEG or force an average reference. Immediately to the right, the user may select predefined frequency bands or enter discrete frequencies for analysis.

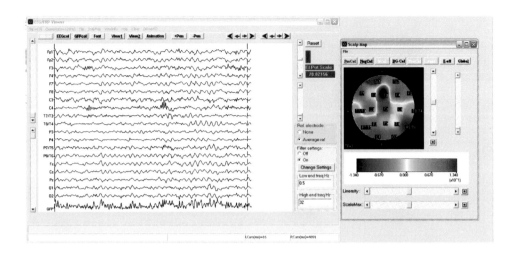

Figure 10: LORETA explorer for EEG/ERP data from LORETA main screen. In the left window is the EEG signal for each electrode. The two signals at the bottom (in blue) are the LORETA global field power curve (GFP) and the local global field power curve (LGFP). Check boxes are available for reference, filter, and band pass settings. The scale can be adjusted for linearity and scaling. By default, each map is displayed relative to its own maximum.

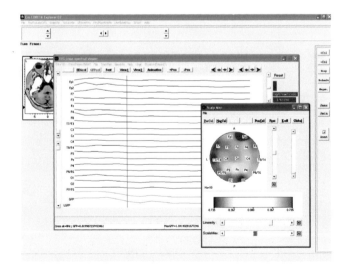

Figure 11: LORETA cross spectra viewer. This module permits the user to view the square root of cross spectra and generators of EEG frequency components. This module is similar to the EEG/ERP viewer in Figure 10 without options, as all information is included in the cross spectra file. An additional function is to select a section of the CRS for analysis (time-domain) and viewing the LORETA. Lower section of the window contains data relative to timeframe (number of seconds), which is important to ERP data.

2.3: Transformation Matrix

The LORETA transformation matrix is calculated using the electrode coordinates created earlier. The signal-to-noise ratio (SNR) is the ratio of the sinusoid power to the noise power (or variance) at the sinusoid frequency. SNR increases as sinusoid power increases at born channels in each epoch. Since the sinusoids have fixed relative phase and amplitude, coherence is proposed to be directly related to SNR (Bendat, 2001). The user may perform the TM manually by simply pressing the go button as shown in Figure 12. Otherwise, the automatic and pseudo-batch options are available. The automatic mode will create a number of automatic TM files with different regularization parameters. The user can view the exact computations in the help file (Gomez & Thatcher, 2001). The edited EEG samples are divided into successive 2-second epochs of 256 time points with Fast Fourier Transform (FFT) cross-spectral analysis (Gomez & Thatcher, 2001). Subsequent analyses depend on the selection and organization of discrete frequency domains to be used. The number of variables can be reduced such that 1 Hz frequency bins can be averaged into x number of frequency bands. The LORETA algorithm computes a T-matrix of current source density according to the Talairach coordinates of the Montreal Neurological Institutes' Magnetic Resonance Imaging average of 305 adult human brains (Lancaster et al., 2000). The diagonal elements of the Hermitian cross-spectral matrix are multiplied by the T-matrix at each frequency domain for each 2-second epoch. The T-matrix is a 3-dimensional matrix of x, y, and z coordinates of the 2,394 7mm^3 grey matter pixels in LORETA.

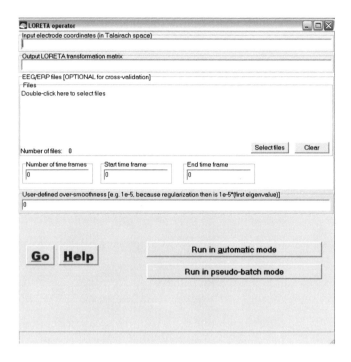

Figure 12: Transformation matrix module. The EEG files listed are for cross-validation and not necessary to create the TM file. The electrode coordinates are used to create the TM. In this example, the timeframes (16) is 16 2s epochs and the start and finish TF equal the number of discrete frequencies to be analyzed in the data set: delta, theta, alpha-1, alpha-2 and beta.

2.4: LORETA Interface and Talairach Atlas

Figure 13 shows the localized current sources for the alpha-2 frequency for a group of 15 subjects. The sources are mapped in Talairach space. The images are orthogonal slices from the brain; from left to right are horizontal, saggital, and coronal views of the brain. The *x* coordinates are negative for the left hemisphere and positive for the right. The *y* coordinates are positive for anterior and negative for posterior locations. The *z* coordinates are positive in superior and negative in ventral locations. The image shows the maximal EEG source for alpha-2 at coordinates **x = 4, y = -81, z = 8**. The positive LORETA values are shown in red and negative values in blue while white indicates zero. The check boxes permit the user to control the scrolling through the time frames. The buttons on the right allow control of colors, maximum or minimum, and map options. The time frames (in the frequency domain) are discrete frequency bands (delta, theta, alpha-1, alpha-2 and beta). One good and simple localization check involves analyzing a subject's eyes-closed EEG for the alpha frequency. In normal subjects, a posterior dominance is shown for alpha that attenuates when the eyes are opened. For more information about the Talairach Atlas visit (http://www.talairach.org/) or see reference (Talairach J, 1988). Additionally, corrections used to transform MNI space to Talairach coordinates may be reviewed in (Brett, Johnsrude, & Owen, 2002) and technical appendices in the LORETA help files can also be utilized.

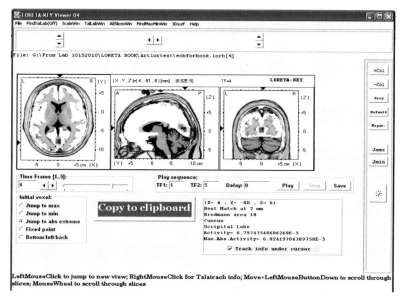

Figure 13: LORETA sources for alpha-2 for cross-spectra in Figure 11.

Figure 14 (next page) shows the LORETA scaling for current source density (CSD) displays. Typically, we choose the higher end of the scale (>.90) to localize the maximum extreme. Lower threshold (actual max or global max) produces more intense color on the map.

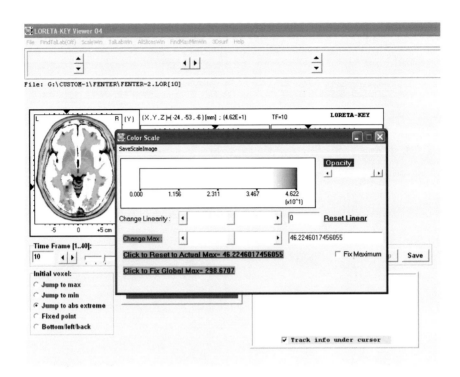

Figure 14: LORETA viewer and scaling options window. With this module, the user can define the scaling of the display. The lower the scaling the more color appears in the map relative to the actual max and global max.

2.5: LORETA Statistics Modules

LORETA utilizes statistical procedures for both ERP (time domain) and EEG (frequency domain) data used in other neuroimaging methodologies. Statistical inferences in the neuroimaging field need to be approached with caution and responsibility. Our current integrative knowledge of regional functions, frequency specificity, functional integration, and network interdependency in the brain is still in its infancy. Thus, many critics of neuroscience focus on the interpretations and inferences made by researchers. In recent years, it is becoming more apparent that localization theory alone does not produce a comprehensive understanding of the brain and the intricacies of interactions between neural modules and networks. Typically, two approaches are taken to analyze brain activation patterns during specific tasks. First, a distributed systems approach examines correlated physiologic components. Second, focal differences are detected based on a specialized, functionally segregated approach.

The statistical tests used in the LORETA program are based on statistical parametric mapping (SPM) (Friston et al., 1990; Friston, Frith, Liddle, & Frackowiak, 1991; Friston et al., 1995). This approach utilizes properties of the general linear model and a design matrix for neurophysiological data. The specific effects (noise or specific activations) are estimated using standard least squares or parameter estimates of the linear model such that the differences in these estimates determine each specific effect. Each contrast computes a t-statistic for each voxel to form the statistical map. The images are then mapped onto a standardized coordinate space to account for differences in brain size and orientation, and the subtracted images are averaged to improve the signal to noise ratio. LORETA implements similar SPM procedures with additional randomization and permutation tests. The tests are performed with a reference distribution obtained from all possible values of the test statistic for all observed data points. Randomization and permutation tests are demonstrated to significantly control for the family wise error rate in multiple hypothesis testing.

The analysis of functional mapping data is typically done on a voxel by voxel basis, producing a statistical image of the differences between conditions or a statistical parametric map. This procedure is designed to account for simultaneous testing of all voxels without an a priori anatomical hypothesis (Fox, 1995; Friston et al., 1990; Friston et al., 1991; Nichols & Holmes, 2002; Petersson, Nichols, Poline, & Holmes, 1999). It needs to be noted that obtaining a sound background in neuroanatomy and neurophysiology is important for making *apriori* hypotheses regarding expected changes during a specific experimental stimulus presentation.

Statistical tests in LORETA are done using either a text file to tell the program where and what files to compare or by entering the files into the provided statistics 'info file' maker (the more user-friendly option). Figure 15 shows the statistics options from the LORETA main screen with numerous options available to the user.

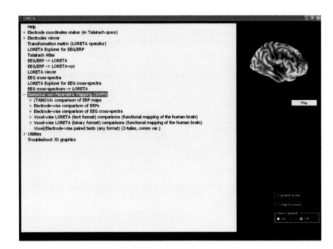

Figure 15: LORETA statistical modules. Options are available for ERP, EEG cross-spectra, and LORETA images.

Figure 16 (next page) shows the statistics 'info file' maker interface. This module is accessible from the utilities option in the main window. The contents of the computer are displayed from left to right. The contents of the selected folder and files can be dragged and dropped into the designated panes (list A or B). In the lower section of the window are the parameters indicating the number of time frames (discrete frequencies), voxels, and time frames/discrete frequencies to be compared. This last designation involves total power, which indicates inclusion of all frequencies, 1 - 5, or a specific discrete frequency 4 - 4 (as shown in figure 15).

Figure 17 (next page) shows the statistical test interface. Listed from the top to the bottom are the parameters to be utilized by the procedure, type of cross-spectra test, ERP/EEG or LORETA, data normalization or log transform (negative values cannot be transformed), test to be performed, data type (LORETA is binary - output from test is text), number of randomizations, and the location of the test-info created in Figure 17 (clicked and selected).

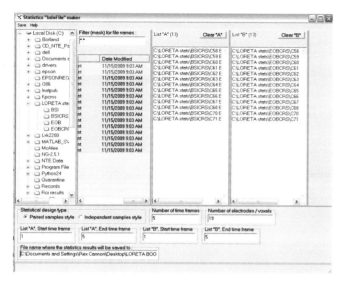

Figure 16: Inputting LORETA statistics into file maker. The four panes across the top from left to right show the computer contents and files within the folder and list A and B (dragged and dropped) to be compared. The spaces at the bottom contain info for the comparison, including the type of test, number of time frames (or discrete frequencies), list A time frames, list B time frames, and finally the file name to be saved.

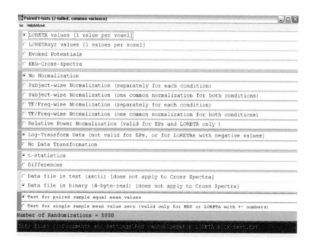

Figure 17: LORETA paired t-test module. With the text file entered from the previous module, the statistics can be computed. The options are available by selecting from a list of options with a click. For the sake of simplicity, the image shows only the basics. This sample compares a visual evaluation of a photograph of a novel female face with eyes-open baseline.

Tests are then conducted between conditions or groups for each time frame or discrete frequency domain. The critical values set for the tests are t < .05 and < .01 and are calculated via randomization procedures (Friston et al., 1990; Friston et al., 1991; Friston et al., 1995). The output of the tests are placed in the folder specified by the user in text format with the extension "-Thresh&Ps.txt." The output of the tests contains exact z-values for the element being contrasted (i.e., EP, LORETA, or CS). It is important to note that users may check specific probabilities associated with the current source density obtained by the tests in particular regions of interest in software modules. It is not always the case that a high z or t level is needed for a significant finding, given the degrees of freedom and parameters of the comparison (Friston et al., 1990; Friston et al., 1991; Friston et al., 1995). Depending on the experimental parameters, typical tests are utilized, e.g., paired t-tests or independent samples t-tests, which are appropriate for these types of data. Figure 18 shows the results of the voxel by voxel-paired t-tests for viewing a novel female face as contrasted to eyes-opened baseline.

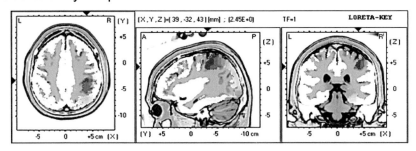

Figure 18: Example set results. The region of increased current source density in the alpha-2 frequency occurs at 39, -32, 43 inferior parietal lobe in the right hemisphere. The t-value 2.45 is significant with 18 degrees of freedom at p = .024.

The region with the maximum increase in current source density between the conditions is shown in the alpha-2 frequency at x = 39, y = -32, z = 43, inferior parietal lobe in the right hemisphere. This area is equivalent to Brodmann area 37 or fusiform region, and it has been shown to be associated with facial recognition or responses to faces in other neuroimaging studies. The t-value of 2.45 is significant with 18 degrees of freedom at p = .024. Importantly, other areas are also increased, such as BA 19, 18, and parieto-temporal regions.

Options exist to extrapolate the current source density and contrast conditions using methods that are more complex (e.g., linear mixed models with repeated measures). It is important to note that the number of samples taken from the subjects does increase the likelihood of interdependence and as such, measures to control this effect are needed

(Cannon et al., 2009; Cannon et al., 2007). It is important to note that the results of the statistical tests are not expressed in standardized values; instead, they indicate within or between group differences. LORETA contains a significant number of tools to permit the user to monitor effectively the change in the EEG and LORETA sources within groups and between groups, as well as the individual patient, which is particularly important for reporting treatment outcomes in neurofeedback training.

2.6: Standardized Low-Resolution Electromagnetic Tomography (sLORETA)

The more recent and accurate release of LORETA is standardized low-resolution electromagnetic tomography or sLORETA. This version also contains exact low-resolution electromagnetic tomography (eLORETA), which provides an exact, error free EEG source localization platform (Pascual-Marqui, 2002; Pascual-Marqui et al., 2002). Figure 19 shows the main welcome page of the sLORETA program. The tabs at the top of the screen show main utilities. Listed from left to right are sLORETA viewer and file explorer, statistical program, help, exit, a PowerPoint tutorial, and finally a module for connectivity analyses.

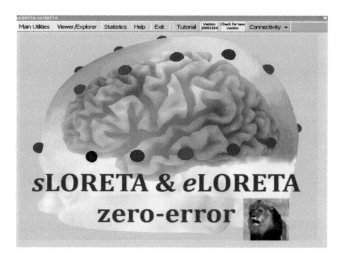

Figure 19: sLORETA/eLORETA main screen. Tabs in the menu bar access each module in the software package.

The user-friendly modules in sLORETA are in tabbed format on the initial screen of the program. The menu contains three basic interfaces in the order in which they are used. In the following sections, I will use examples to cover each. The first is the main utility module, which consists of conversion of ERP/EEG data in the same fashion as using LORETA, setting up electrodes, cross spectra, transformation matrix, and sLORETA images. Second, I will cover the viewer interface, which is more complex compared to its predecessor. Lastly, I will cover the statistical modules in sLORETA, the testing, and the results.

The sLORETA main utilities screen utilizes a tabbed format to access different modules for converting EEG/ERP data for use by the sLORETA program. Figure 20 shows the sLORETA main screen with tabs in the top right section.

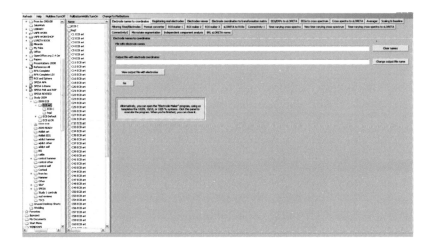

Figure 20: sLORETA main utilities screen. From left to right are the contents of the computer, the specific folder selected, and the contents and the tabs for the different modules for use in sLORETA.

As in LORETA, the first step is to create an electrode coordinate (EC) file. This is the first tab on the menu bar. Once selected, a new interface opens as shown in Figure 21.

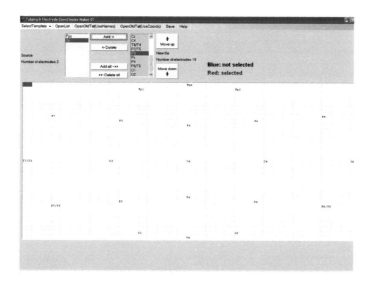

Figure 21: sLORETA electrode coordinates maker. In the top left is the tab for a preset template 10/20, 10/10, or 10/5 system, respectively. As shown in the image, the selected electrode is red and deselected electrodes remain blue. After selecting the appropriate electrodes, the user saves the coordinate file by clicking the save button in the menu bar and providing a name for the file.

The user can import a text file or create an EC file by clicking the box near the bottom with the text in the center. If 10/20 is selected, the user can click the 'select all' option. The user is advised that the electrodes should match the montage with which the data was collected. For example, on the Electrocap, there is not an Oz electrode: therefore, it should be removed from the coordinate file. It is important that the electrode coordinates file be synchronized with the collection device in order to prevent errors. In Figure 22, from left to right, are the contents of the computer (files that can be accessed by drag and drop), with the specific contents of the folder selected in the next slot. It is important for the user to organize files that will be analyzed in folders with nomenclature that is easily remembered and identifiable. Over the course of analyses, the number of files will increase; therefore, it is helpful to use a systematic approach with appropriately organized data. Compared to the original program, the sLORETA program contains additional analytical tools. Since this manuscript is dedicated to basic concepts, it will not address more complex procedures; however, modules are available to conduct the analysis of functional connectivity and other more complex procedures (Cannon, 2009).

2.7: Transformation Matrix

Figure 22 shows the transformation matrix module. The electrode coordinates file is entered in the space provided (drag and drop). Afterwards, the user can select available options. The optional categories are regularization and the specific tomography (sLORETA or eLORETA). After selecting the mode of regularization, the output will place four files with different parameters (signal to noise ratios of 1, 10, 100, and 1000) in the main operating folder. This module converts the electrode coordinates to sLORETA TM. The electrode coordinates file (has sxyz file name, for example, 19.sxyz) will be entered in the first space provided. The TM file is automatically named with the TM extension (for example spinv.). After entering the file and selecting regularization and the specific tomography options, the user can click the go button. The TM output will be placed in the same folder that contains the electrode coordinates file. It will be needed for subsequent modules.

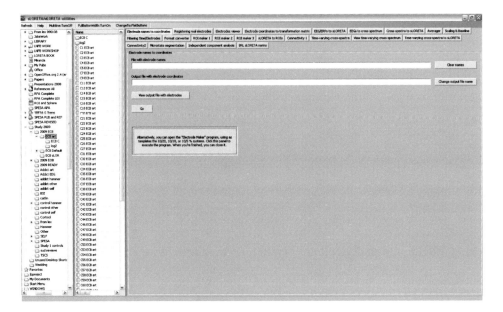

Figure 22: sLORETA transformation matrix module. This module converts the electrode coordinates to sLORETA TM. The electrode coordinates file is entered in the first space (has sxyz file name, e.g., 19.sxyz). The TM file is automatically named with the TM extension (spinv). Options are available for regularization and the zero-error tomography (sLORETA or eLORETA). Once the file is entered and options are selected, the user clicks the go button. The TM output will be placed in the folder where the electrode coordinates file is stored.

Figure 23 shows the module used to convert EEG to cross-spectra and cross-spectra to sLORETA (.slor) files. In essence, this module has similar features to the cross spectra maker in LORETA only with a different interface. The user can simply drag and drop the EEG files into the large space provided, check the appropriate mode of operation, and enter the number of electrodes, number of time frames, and sampling rate. Additionally, the user can check the average reference, choose the frequency range, or provide a discrete frequency range. Finally, the user enters the file name for the cross spectra output and clicks go. The output files will be placed in the designated folder with the EEG data by default. The output file for the cross spectra will have a CRSS extension.

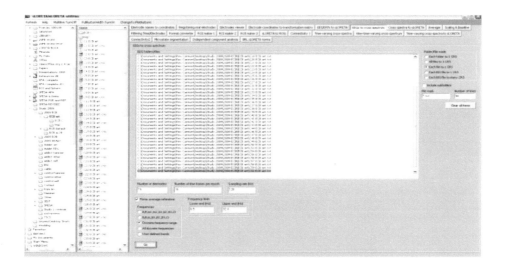

Figure 23: sLORETA EEG to cross spectra module. The EEG files are dragged and dropped into the provided space. The data specific parameters are then entered: number of electrodes, number of time frames per epoch, sampling rate, frequency domain selection. In this example, the frequency range of interest contains inclusively 0.5 - 32.0 Hz; given the specs, this will equate to five discrete frequency bands. In the top right corner, there are options for the type of output. In this example, dataset one, CRS for each file (or each subject in this condition), will be output.

Figure 24 (next page) shows the module for converting the CRSS files to sLORETA. The user simply drags and drops the CRSS files into the provided space, selects the time frames or frequency range to be analyzed, drags and drops the TM file into the provided space, and clicks go.

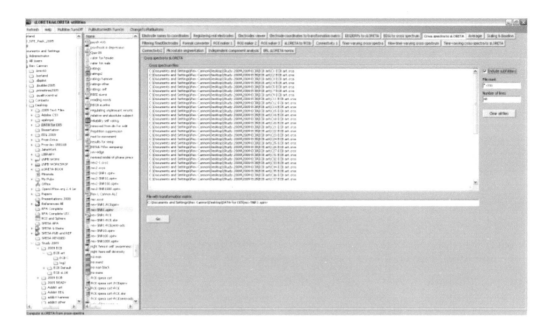

Figure 24: sLORETA cross spectra to sLORETA module. The CRSS files created in Figure 23 are dragged and dropped into the provided space. The transformation matrix file is entered into the required space and the go button is clicked. These files will be placed in the same folder as the CRS files and will be labeled with the extension slor.

Figure 25 shows the sLORETA viewer for an eyes-closed resting baseline recording. The sLORETA viewer contains several components for viewing the data. Image (A) shows the global field power/loreta max, (B) shows the MNI maps for the sources of EEG, (C) shows the file explorer and the sLORETA file selected, and (D) shows the 3D cortex of EEG sources. These panes can be organized in any manner on the screen; similarly, the sLORETA maps can be saved as bitmap images for publication and other purposes. The viewer will be revisited again in the statistics section.

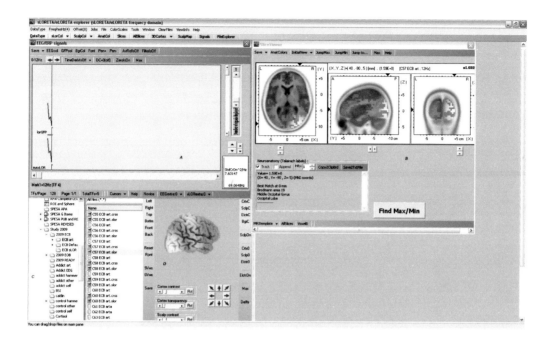

Figure 25: sLORETA viewer. Each sectional component within this caption has its own window. The top left shows the global field power and maximum current source density. Depending on the discrete frequency, range is the length of the lorGFP signal. Clicking the red arrows will feed through the time frames and change the sLORETA map accordingly. The top left shows horizontal, saggital, and axial views of the brain at MNI coordinates 40, -90, 5. This image shows sources for the alpha-2 frequency 10 - 12 Hz in an eyes-closed condition. The arrows under each image allow for progression through the map in the current orientation. The text below the image shows the value at the voxel, coordinates, spatial resolution, and Brodmann area/anatomical label. The bottom left shows the file explorer with the current file highlighted. Finally, (D) shows the 3D cortex. This last map can be rotated with the red arrows in the window. Additional options are available to change the features of the map.

2.8: Statistics in sLORETA

The sLORETA program has statistical modules presented in the tabbed format, as shown in earlier figures. It contains several pages of user-defined options that progress to the final statistical comparison. The first option is the data type with ERP, sLORETA, sLORETA-XYZ, and cross spectrum, measures of dependence, or time varying log-spectra. The user analyzing ERP data has different options to select from, including average reference, number of electrodes, and number of time frames. Computation of an average reference and the implications are discussed in detail (Pascual-Marqui & Lehmann, 1993a, 1993b). LORETA's current density estimation is the same for any choice of common cranial reference (Pascual-Marqui et al., 1999; Pascual-Marqui, 1999).

The next screen in the statistical procedures is the data normalization or scaling for the data. The available options are none, time-frame/frequency wise, subject-wise, or electrode/voxel wise (relative power type). The time-frame/frequency wise normalization is a normalization of each image or an image wise scaling. The subject wise option normalizes the total power over all images of each subject and finally the electrode/voxel-wise option normalizes the time signal or the spectra at each voxel. The next screen lists the types of tests to be conducted. The options are paired groups (A = B), independent groups (A = B), paired group (A - A2) = (B - B2), independent group (A - A2) = (B - B2), regression, single group with external independent variable and finally, regression paired contrast (A1 - A2) regressed on external independent variable (i.e., psychometric test scores).

The next screen contains a baseline correction option that will be used with ERP (or time specific) data. Figure 26 illustrates the selection of files to be compared. The figure shows, from left to right, the contents of the computer and selected folder, the next frame shows the contents of the selected folder, and finally list A and B to be compared. As mentioned in the caption, for a within-subjects comparison, it is imperative that list A corresponds directly to list B. Once the files are entered and checked for accuracy, the user clicks the next button. If the cross spectra - EEG step was performed correctly, all sLOR files should be the same size. Any discrepancy will result in error or a convergence failure.

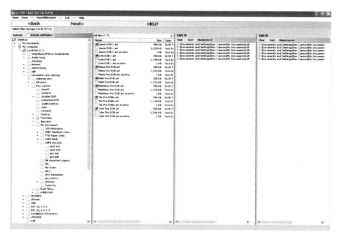

Figure 26: sLORETA statistics file selection window. The image from left to right shows the folders in the computer, the files within the selected folder, and files dragged into list A and B. This is a paired comparison within groups, evaluating an image of a novel other face compared to eyes-opened baseline. It is important that for list A to be directly synchronized with list B.

The next screen (figure 27 - next page) lists the specific test details with the following options: all tests for all time frames or frequencies, 1 single average test for a specified time frame interval, or multiple tests for each time frame or frequency in a specified interval. Here we need to remind the user that the frequencies are assigned to a time frame in the earlier conversion process: for the data in this example, TF 1 = delta, TF 2 = theta, TF 3 = alpha-1, TF 4 = alpha-2, and TF 5 = beta. In this example, we choose all tests for each time frame or frequency in a specified interval and then click next. In this example, we would chose data 1 - 5 for list A and 1 - 5 for list B, since we are interested in frequency specific changes that occur between the stimulus and baseline. The intervals can be specific to one frequency by only selecting the time frame for that specific frequency, e.g., list A 1 - 1 and list B 1 - 1. The next screen provides options for selecting the types of tests. Figure 27 shows the options. For the example data set, we choose a t-test on log-transformed data with spatial smoothing at 1 and 5,000 data randomizations. The file is named _otherbook_ and then the program progresses to the next screen, which simply provides an interactive button to perform the test. The duration of the test and drain on computer resources depends on the number of files, time frames, and other properties of the data to be analyzed. Typically, the test computes in rapid fashion.

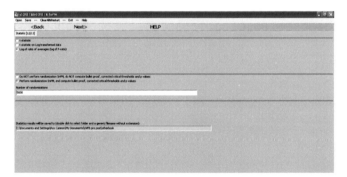

Figure 27: Time frame interval options.

Figure 28 shows the results for the comparison in the alpha-2 frequency domain (TF 4). The window contains the file folder, the sLORETA global field power, sLORETA maximum, the MNI atlas, and the 3D cortical map. The statistical output consists of a text file with the test information and a text file with the thresholds and significance levels thereof.

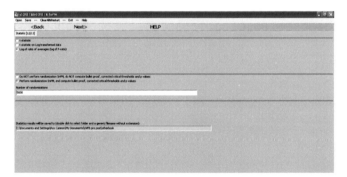

Figure 28: sLORETA statistics options window. The specific tests are selected in this window. The available options are t-statistic, t-statistic on log transformed data, log of ration of average (log of F-ratio), randomization, corrected critical thresholds (typically 5,000 data randomizations are used in neuroimaging data), and finally the name of the file to be saved. For the example data, we selected the t-statistic on log-transformed data with 5,000 data randomizations and named the results otherbook. To select the log-transformed option, a window is added for the smoothing option. Since we want optimal localization with normalized data, we set the smoothing to 1.

Figure 29 (next page) shows the screen that appears during the statistical calculations. Typically, the procedures run rapidly; however, depending on the size and complexity of the data, the statistical procedures may run more slowly and drain computer resources for a short time.

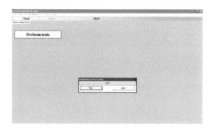

Figure 29: sLORETA window during the statistical calculations.

The exceedence proportion test reports a collection of threshold values and associated probabilities. In the context of neuroimaging data, exceedingly high number of data points exists for each subject for each comparison; thus, it may not be necessary to obtain a high value to indicate a significant finding. The exceedence proportion test may also indicate significance when voxel by voxel tests do not. For more specific information about the exceedence proportion tests and significance levels, see references (Friston et al., 1990; Friston et al., 1991). To check the reported significance levels for voxels of interest, the value can be entered into any probability calculator with the correct degrees of freedom. To control for type I error in a strong sense, it is prudent to check voxels of interest as there may be a type II error. In Figure 30, the value of the test is 2.50 with 22 degrees of freedom, showing that a probability of t for a two-tailed test is .022. Thus, for example, the maximum increase in current source density for evaluating the face of a novel female occurs in the right parietal lobe, specifically the precuneus, at x = 25, y = -60, z = 65. The minimum difference in current source density between conditions is at Brodmann Area 9, middle frontal gyrus (x = -45, y = 25, z = 40). The t value is 1.81 with the probability of t = .08. Other test results are observed by scrolling with the arrow through the global field power window for each TF.

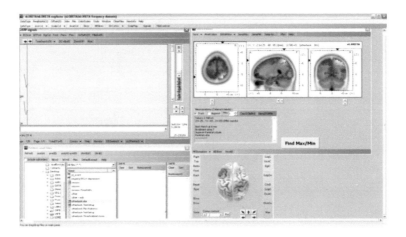

Figure 30: sLORETA statistical results. The blue shows decreased CSD between conditions, red shows increased CSD and yellow indicates maximum increase.

2.9: Summary

The modules in LORETA and s/eLORETA are run in a specific sequence in order to localize the EEG sources. First, the electrode coordinates must be defined according to the EEG recording device. Second, the electrode coordinates are utilized to create the transformation matrix of the cross spectra with signal to noise ratios. Third, the EEG files are entered into the LORETA interface and cross-spectral matrices are then computed. Fourth, the cross-spectral matrices or EEG files are entered into the LORETA or sLORETA/ eLORETA conversion (e.g., EEG sources). Statistical analyses can then be run for the time domain or frequency domain. Statistical images can then be interpreted for publication. Certain simple checks are available for LORETA, with the most obvious being the alpha frequency (7.5 - 12.0 Hz) for eyes-closed resting condition that should appear in posterior regions and attenuate during eyes-opened baseline, barring any known psychopathologic or neurologic condition that may affect this prominent feature of the EEG. Similarly, artifacts (physical or mechanical) may produce anomalies in the EEG source localization, which are typically easily seen in the raw EEG data. LORETA and the standardized (sLORETA) and exact (eLORETA) versions are validated as accurate. They provide an inexpensive, non-invasive, potentially less anxiety evoking method to investigate the human brain in intricate detail, presenting exciting options for neurophysiology and neuroscience research and clinical practice.

CHAPTER 3

Clinical Applications of Quantitative EEG (QEEG) and LORETA

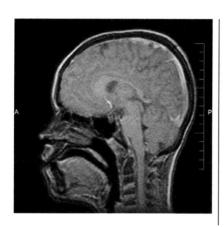
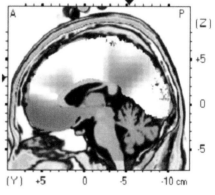

CHAPTER 3

Clinical Applications of Quantitative EEG (qEEG) and LORETA

Quantitative EEG (qEEG) comprises computerized imaging and statistical procedures to aid in the detection of abnormal patterns associated with specific pathological conditions and normative patterns found in different cognitive and affective conditions (Bjork et al., 2008; Castellanos et al., 1996; Kaiser, 2007; Pascual-Montano, Taylor, Winkler, Pascual-Marqui, & Carazo, 2002; Winterer et al., 1998). As such, qEEG is a direct signature of neural activity and provides ideal temporal resolution in the millisecond time domain (Coburn et al., 2006; Hughes & John, 1999). Additionally, qEEG and LORETA provide a method to evaluate the brain mechanisms associated with the experience of a stimulus, such that the moment of decision or time locked event associated with a stimuli is important. Yet, the state of subjective changes during the processing of stimuli may indeed prove more interesting and informative (Cannon, 2009; Cannon, Baldwin, & Lubar, 2008). Both qEEG and LORETA are important methodologies for demonstrating the direct associations between psychiatric conditions and symptoms associated with neurologic functions (Hughes & John, 1999) as well as monitoring pharmacological effects (Saletu et al., 1997) and treatment outcomes (Czobor & Volavka, 1991; Prichep et al., 2002).

Additionally, due to its noninvasive properties, qEEG affords the opportunity to examine the brain's electrical activity during longer periods in variable experimental conditions (Cannon, 2009; Cannon, Baldwin, & Lubar, 2008). Combined with LORETA source localization, qEEG proves to be an invaluable tool in both research and clinical settings. Importantly, in current practice qEEG is not endorsed by the American Medical Association for diagnostic purposes except for the conditions of epilepsy and sleep disturbances. However, I can affirm with confidence that this will change in coming years.

This chapter briefly reviews research findings in normal populations and psychiatric disorders. It is important to note that qEEG and LORETA can be a very powerful adjunct to other, more established techniques, such as fMRI or PET. The benefit to using these types of measures in unison with LORETA is that combined, they facilitate the discovery of frequency specific functions in the human brain relative to specific behaviors.

The validity and reliability of qEEG has been an area of concentrated study. A large number (>100) of peer-reviewed articles in PubMed demonstrate the reliability and validity of qEEG methods (Corsi-Cabrera, Galindo-Vilchis, del-Rio-Portilla, Arce, & Ramos-Loyo, 2007; Corsi-Cabrera, Guevara, Arce, & Ramos, 1996; Corsi-Cabrera, Solis-Ortiz, & Guevara, 1997; Guevara, Lorenzo, Arce, Ramos, & Corsi-Cabrera, 1995). Therefore, many arguments against the computerized analyses of EEG may not carry much validity, especially when considering that no existing studies published to date show significant reliability of non-computerized analysis of the EEG signal (Hughes & John, 1999).

The spectral analysis of the qEEG is suggested to be clinically useful for revealing additional signs of brain dysfunction in individual patients, and it is considered a valuable research tool for revealing statistical differences between groups (Coutin-Churchman et al., 2003). Notably, the apriori fundamental elements of learning and behavior occur neurologically, and they are certainly very important for understanding normative and psychopathological functions. Alterations of the EEG power spectra are more likely to occur with a high statistical significance in certain disorders. Although this association is not deterministic and several dissimilar or even contradictory patterns can occur within a given diagnostic category, it is important to consider carefully the symptomology, behavioral measures, and cortical indications. Hence, it is very important to consider the clinical and research potential of qEEG computer assisted diagnostic procedures to perform accurately, in some cases with the fundamental acknowledgement, that only one source of information is not adequate for diagnostic purposes (John, 1989; John, Prichep, Fridman, & Easton, 1988). PET and fMRI have superior spatial resolution, yet these methods only provide the 'where' of brain, whereas qEEG and LORETA may provide important knowledge into the 'what' of the brain (Cannon et al., 2009). This section could be a book in itself; therefore, the reviews will be brief and specific to neuroimaging, qEEG, and LORETA findings in Depression and Anxiety (including OCD), Substance Use Disorders (SUD), and Attention Deficit/Hyperactivity Disorder (ADHD). This chapter will also review research studies on normal cognitive, executive, attention and self-affect regulation (self-regulation) processes.

3.1: Major Depressive Disorder

Depression is one of the most studied disorders in human psychopathology. The use of neurophysiology and hormonal indices as a measure of emotion (stress and negative affect) is based on the assumption that different emotions are associated with distinct patterns of physiological responses. Although the neural patterns of autonomic activity associated with different emotions are not well understood, considerable evidence for physiological response patterns indicates that autonomic activity is differentiated along multiple evaluative dimensions of emotion (Averill, 1983; Dienstbier, Hillman, Lehnhoff, Hillman, & Valkenaar, 1975; Goldstein, 1968; Lang, 1979; Lang, Kozak, Miller, Levin,

& McLean, 1980; Rosenblatt & Thickstun, 1977). The use of qEEG and LORETA has provided a rather large, important contribution to our understanding of depression and the associative involvement of brain regions, neurotransmitters, and functional connectivity patterns.

In recent years, a growing interest has developed regarding the role of the prefrontal cortex (PFC) in stress and depression and the possible influences of the PFC on the stress hormone cortisol. Thus, in discussing depression, I will also include references to stress, cortisol, and cognitive components, as combinations of these factors contribute to the etiology of depressive disorders. The hypothalamic-pituitary-adrenal axis (HPA) and the neurochemical consequences of stress are well studied. Acute stress is shown to activate the sympathetic nervous system in part through the release of adrenalin and noradrenalin. The HPA axis and the stress hormone cortisol are involved in the long term adaptation to stress (Sapolsky, 2004). Increased levels of the adrenergic neurotransmitters are manifested in behavioral reactions in the form of irritability, arousal, and the startle response. Cortisol has been shown to regulate its own release via a negative feedback loop in the CNS. In order to facilitate this, it binds to specific receptors throughout the limbic system, including the hippocampus, amygdala, and prefrontal cortex (Feldman & Weidenfeld, 1995; Herman & Cullinan, 1997). These adrenergic increases play a role in posttraumatic stress disorder (PTSD) in children and adults (Schwarz & Perry, 1994). Chronic or long-term exposure to stressful stimuli activates the HPA axis, which causes a release of cortisol. It is thought that stress is a subjective experience, viz., that what is stressful to one individual may not be stressful to another. Similarly, an event that induces stress at one instant in time may not produce the same effect in the next instant (Thornton & Andersen, 2006). In general, cortisol is a favorable hormone that is important in the regulation of physiological systems. Cortisol plays a role in the regulation of metabolism by mobilizing energy resources for the body. However, elevated levels of cortisol are connected to depression (Holsboer, 2001), diminished immunity (Dickerson &

Kemeny, 2004), hypertension, and diabetes (McEwen, 1998). Cortisol secretion operates in conjunction with circadian rhythms, with peaking levels in the morning and lower levels at night.

Numerous regions in the cortex, including the hypothalamus, hippocampus, pituitary gland, brain-stem, prefrontal, and limbic regions, are associated with this stress-induction and stress-reduction processes (Figueiredo, Bodie, Tauchi, Dolgas, & Herman, 2003; Figueiredo, Bruestle, Bodie, Dolgas, & Herman, 2003; Herman, Figueiredo, et al., 2003). Neurons in the hippocampus are particularly susceptible to prolonged exposure to increased cortisol and deleterious effects are observed in memory functions. Similar effects are also shown in the prefrontal cortices, and this combination of effects is associated with the manifestation of depressive symptoms (LeDoux, 1998; LeDoux & Gorman, 2001). Stress leads to subjective anxiety, endocrine activation of HPA axis, and cardiovascular changes (Sinha, Catapano, & O'Malley, 1999). Recent advancements in functional and structural neuroimaging methods have increased the potential to investigate directly these regulatory networks in humans. Several notable studies provide evidence for regulatory roles of the hippocampus, amygdale, and prefrontal cortex in the human stress response (Dagher, Tannenbaum, Hayashi, Pruessner, & McBride, 2009; Dedovic, Duchesne, Andrews, Engert, & Pruessner, 2009; Dedovic et al., 2005; Pruessner et al., 2008; Pruessner et al., 1997; Pruessner, Hellhammer, Pruessner, & Lupien, 2003; Soliman et al., 2008; Wang et al., 2007; Wang et al., 2005). Importantly, according to recent data, brainstem nuclei play an important role in cortisol regulation, considering that neuroimaging studies examining neural changes in response to physical stressors are scant in current literature.

Research has shown that the effects of early experiences can influence cortisol levels permanently and negatively. For example, animals that display a heightened stress response throughout the lifespan do so as a result of possible negative effects on the hippocampal formation and because of the ability of the hippocampus to perform efficiently when special effort is necessary (LeDoux & Gorman, 2001). Cortisol levels have also been shown to be elevated in children raised in orphanages or with insecure attachment to caregivers (Gunnar, 1998). EEG studies with nonhuman primates have reported that right PFC EEG activity was associated with higher cortisol levels (Kalin, Larson, Shelton, & Davidson, 1998; Kalin, Shelton, & Davidson, 2000). Similarly, 6-month old infants with extreme right frontal EEG amplitude at rest had higher cortisol levels overall compared to infants with extreme right frontal EEG during a withdrawal task. Thus, it was concluded that the right prefrontal cortex plays an important role in withdrawal-related emotional behavior and fearful temperament (Buss et al., 2003; Kalin, Shelton, & Barksdale, 1987).

A high percentage of depressed patients show increased patterns of EEG alpha and or theta power over the prefrontal cortices during baseline or emotional tasks relative to the type and degree of depressive symptoms (John et al., 1988; Pollock & Schneider, 1990). Additionally, interhemispheric asymmetry is often found in depressed patients with alpha power being greater over the right frontal regions while the opposite effect is seen in parietal cortices (Henriques & Davidson, 1991). Questions remain, however, regarding the role of right frontal EEG alpha activity and its relationship to depression as this alpha asymmetry finding continues to present with additional EEG sources, which adds to the concept of distributed networks functioning in both normal populations and psychiatric syndromes. LORETA has been employed to evaluate treatment response, interhemispheric asymmetry, and cognitive processes among depressive patients (Davidson, Pizzagalli, Nitschke, & Putnam, 2002; Flor-Henry, Lind, & Koles, 2004; Lubar et al., 2003; Mientus et al., 2002; Pizzagalli et al., 2001; Pizzagalli, Nitschke, et al., 2002).

Researchers using variable resolution electrical tomography (VARETA) showed that depressed patients have increased percentages of EEG sources in both hemispheres, favoring the right hemisphere. Abnormal current source density was also observed in dorsolateral prefrontal, superior parietal, and precentral gyri (Ricardo-Garcell et al., 2009). Research has demonstrated that the right prefrontal cortex and right limbic regions show an increase in alpha and beta activity during anger memory reclamation and during the evaluation of self and self-in-experience when the experience is perceived as negative. Interestingly, overlap in regional activity occurs during the evaluation of practical joking and humor (Cannon et al., 2008; Cannon, Lubar, Clements, Harvey, & Baldwin, 2008; Cannon, Lubar, Thornton, Wilson, & Congedo, 2004).

It may very well be that rather than one regional focus, research may benefit by considering the possibility of distributed networks in the etiology of depressive disorders (Cannon, 2009; Dedovic et al., 2009). A recent review questioned the role of frontal EEG asymmetry in depression and anxiety, emphasizing especially the lack of stability across studies, including reference site, frequency of interest, location of interest, and psychological indices used to measure the emotional state (i.e., depression inventory, etc.) (Thibodeau, Jorgensen, & Kim, 2006). These areas require clarification and the methods discussed in this manuscript offer solutions to control for this lack of consistency across studies. Evaluating psychological variables and comparing them to a "resting state" may not be the most accurate method to observe the state of interest. It is more interesting to record the individuals in the assessment condition and evaluate spectral power distributions and LORETA activity in these conditions. This is an area of intense interest to the author as well as a more practical procedure for making inferences about location and symptomology. Moreover, stress indices, such as salivary cortisol, can correlate with LORETA in specific tasks or assessment conditions in order to compliment the subjective understanding of the state condition (Cannon, 2009; Cannon, Baldwin, & Lubar, 2008).

Studies suggest that the etiology of depression is more biologically based; however, certain implications suggest that it also relates to psychoimmunological, neurophysiological, and internal (real or imagined) stress response processes. Depression is associated with negative cognitive processes, including hopelessness as well as a dysfunctional view of the world and the individual's place in it (Hammen, 2003). Additional characteristics of depression include loss of enjoyable activity interests (anhedonia), worthlessness, low self-esteem, negative self-image, negative self-efficacy, and external locus of control or a negative view of internal locus of control, i.e., individuals feel responsible for everything bad that happens and hold a negative view of the world (Davidson, Jackson, & Kalin, 2000; Davidson, Putnam, & Larson, 2000).

Recent research by Pizzagalli and colleagues (2007) found correlations among the delta frequency, three regions of interest in the anterior cingulate gyrus (BA 24, 25, and 32), and ratings of Anhedonia. Studies have also demonstrated that the anterior insular cortex in the left hemisphere shows significant volume reductions in patients with current and remittent depression. The anterior insula is proposed to be involved in intereoceptive processes. Additionally, it is active during most functional imaging tasks (Craig, 2009a, 2009b; Ravindran et al., 2009; Takahashi et al., 2010; Yao, Wang, Lu, Liu, & Teng, 2009), especially during emotion and awareness of self and others. Importantly, there are clear functional distinctions between anterior and posterior insula, one of the more interesting of these differences is that the posterior insula is proposed to monitor the feelings associated with the physical body and the integration of this process with other affective and cognitive functions (Craig, 2009a, 2009b). A recent comparison in acutely depressed patients indicated a greater cerebral blood flow increase in the anterior insular cortex during experimentally induced sadness in remitted depressed subjects vulnerable to relapse (Liotti, Mayberg, McGinnis, Brannan, & Jerabek, 2002).This offers evidence that insular cortex abnormalities are intricately involved in the underlying disease processes of MDD. Postmortem studies have also shown cytoarchitectural abnormalities in the antero-ventral insula without anomalous trends in posterior insula, further suggesting that regional insular cortex abnormalities, particularly in the anterior portion, may relate to the neurobiology of major mood disorders (Beckmann & Jakob, 1991; Pennington, Dicker, Dunn, & Cotter,

2008; Pennington, Dicker, Hudson, & Cotter, 2008). The insular cortex is important for monitoring and treating depressive symptoms and is, along with the anterior cingulate, trained and tracked by the methods discussed in this text.

The cognitive model of emotional disorders suggests that the interpretation of events influences both the emotional and behavioral responses to those events. Moreover, it is suggested that beliefs and experiential information determine perception and interpretation of events (Beck, 2008; Beck & Rush, 1985). Beck and associates described a model of emotional disorders in which schemata are formed, and these sets of beliefs and assumptions related to self are suggested to be encoded with emotional material (Beck, 1964; Beck, Hollon, Young, Bedrosian, & Budenz, 1985).

Cognitive theory suggests that some programs are genetically determined, which results in observable behavior patterns, which are proposed to be influenced by cognitive processing, emotive valence, self-regulation, and motivation (Davidson, 2000; Davidson, Jackson, et al., 2000; Davidson, Putnam, et al., 2000; Davidson & Slagter, 2000). These schemata (programs) are reported to influence automatic processes, including affective, perceptive, and behavioral responses that result from evolutionary patterns in animals and humans (Davidson, 2004). Young (1990) proposed that early life experiences and relationships with others influence the development of early maladaptive schemas (EMS). These EMS are suggested to influence self-identity and are maintained, developed, and elaborated on throughout the lifespan (Young, 1990). Moreover, these schemata influence the development of common themes, such as security, autonomy, gratification, self-control, and self-expression, all of which are vital to the development of a functionally integrated self. EMS can cause distress in the individual and, more interestingly, changing or confronting these core beliefs can result in marked distress (Young, 1990). It is proposed that activation of these maladaptive schemata evokes intense negative emotions. Another operational use of schemata involves synaptic or dendritic pruning processes that form in the brain and through which information is filtered. This filter defines the information as positive, negative, fear evoking, or initiating aggressive action (Cannon, Baldwin, & Lubar, 2008; Smythies & Sykes, 1966).

Females are two-times more likely to suffer from depression compared to males; however, it is suggested that males are less likely to seek psychiatric help than are females. Additionally, males suffering from depression are often diagnosed with comorbid substance abuse disorders (Marcus et al., 2005). Associations between cortisol patterns and personality have been observed in early childhood, specifically, among preschool boys. Less labile daily cortisol slopes were associated with negative affect, sadness, and shyness (Dettling, Gunnar, & Donzella, 1999). Similarly, increased social fear was shown to predict flatter diurnal cortisol slopes among preschool boys and girls (Watamura, Donzella, Alwin, & Gunnar, 2003). Other research has shown no differences among adolescent participants in cortisol levels during a social stress test (Bouma, Riese, Ormel, Verhulst, & Oldehinkel, 2009). In addition, research with young participants has shown that levels of self-esteem and locus of control predicted the cortisol stress response and only participants with low self-esteem showed a significant cortisol release in response to the task (Pruessner, Hellhammer, & Kirschbaum, 1999).

Studies report that the stress response initiates increased glucocorticoid levels in the brain and that metatoxic levels of cortisol can cause neuronal damage to specific structures involved in the interpretation of stress, especially the hippocampus (Sala et al., 2004). Of particular note is the finding that hippocampal lesions are shown to ablate the cortisol stress response in humans. This suggests that the role of hippocampus in memory, learning, and emotion is vital to both reactive and autonomic adaptive functions. Neuroimaging studies have shown a decreased hippocampal volume in patients suffering from MDD compared to normal controls (Frodl et al., 2006; Neumeister et al., 2005; Rosso, 2005). LORETA provides the potential to monitor prefrontal regions as well as the insular cortices, hippocampal activity, and numerous other regions implicated in depressive disorders. Treatment induced cortical changes can be monitored with qEEG methods, including neurofeedback protocols as well as group and individual therapy. As such, treatment effects might be determined with contrasts between pre and post measures, or several measures over time.

3.2: Anxiety Disorders

Anxiety is characterized by a negative emotional state mediated by neuronal mechanisms also involved in panic disorder, specifically in the form of anticipatory anxiety. Panic disorder is proposed to consist of three primary psychological components. These components include acute attacks, anticipatory anxiety, and phobic avoidance, and they are suggested to involve the brainstem, limbic system, and prefrontal cortex in a functional network system (Isotani et al., 2001; Milad & Rauch, 2007; Nitschke et al., 2009; Nowak & Marczynski, 1981; Pizzagalli, Nitschke, et al., 2002; Smit, Posthuma, Boomsma, & De Geus, 2007; Thibodeau et al., 2006). The prefrontal cortex plays a critical role in self-regulatory processes and is also proposed to function as a mediator of anxiety and other mood disorders, given its intimate connections with both limbic and brain stem regions (Isotani et al., 2001).

In modernity, the majority of stress that individuals in western cultures experience is more likely a result of psychosocial factors as opposed to life-threatening events that can be more detrimental due to long-term habituation and sensitization of the central nervous system and subsequent dysregulation of homeostasis (wisdom of the body). The brain-activation patterns associated with startle, anger, and fear may still take place during a stress-evoking situation, such as a test or job interview (Wang et al., 2005). These neural patterns associated with stress have been modeled by using the performance of an impromptu speech (McEwen, 2000a, 2000b). Recent data indicate that ventral right prefrontal cortex is specifically associated with psychological stress and that the stress-related activity persists even beyond the stress-task period into a resting baseline (Wang et al., 2005).

Substantial evidence shows that self-affect regulation and emotion relate to functional prefrontal mechanisms (Bruder, Fong, et al., 1997; Bruder, Stewart, et al., 1997; Davidson, 2004; Davidson, Kalin, & Shelton, 1993; Pizzagalli, Lehmann, et al., 2002; Pizzagalli, Nitschke, et al., 2002; Pizzagalli, Sherwood, Henriques, & Davidson, 2005; Tomarken, Davidson, & Henriques, 1990). Whether this pertains to regional specific asymmetry or disruptions within distributed networks involving prefrontal regions is an area of concentrated effort (Cannon, 2009). Research suggests that the anterior cingulate gyrus, in conjunction with prefrontal cortices, limbic structures, and the insula, plays an important role in several psychiatric syndromes. Compared to healthy controls, participants with generalized social anxiety disorder exhibited enhanced bilateral amygdala and insula reactivity to negative rather than neutral images. The extent of amygdala activation correlated with social anxiety severity, whereas the extent of insula activation correlated with trait anxiety, which may also be attributed to threat assessment processing (Shah, Klumpp, Angstadt, Nathan, & Phan, 2009). A prominent panic attacks theory suggests that they occur because of an abnormally sensitive (or perhaps hyperactive) fear network, which includes the prefrontal cortex, insula, thalamus, amygdala, as well as projections from the amygdala to the brainstem and hypothalamus (Gorman, Kent, Sullivan, & Coplan, 2000).

Inverse associations between prefrontal activity and cortisol release (Taylor et al., 2008; Wang et al., 2005) may suggest that the ventrolateral PFC plays a role in providing experiential or genetically encoded data that activate the control of the cortisol release. Although the ventrolateral PFC has scarce projections to the hippocampus, it has extensive connections to the ventromedial prefrontal cortices that are implicated also in the default network of the brain (Peterson et al., 2009). This mechanism could allow ventrolateral PFC to counteract the decrease in activity in orbital and medial PFC areas related to stress processing. Inadequate levels of self-affect-control may be associated with prolonged increased cortisol secretion in association with the anterior cingulate and anterior insular cortices. This would be supported by findings reporting increased ventrolateral PFC activity linked to the lasting effect of stress and increased cortisol secretion (Wang et al., 2005).

AC activity varies considerably across anxiety studies. The AC plays an important role in error monitoring and regulating adaptive behaviors in response to environmental cues (Bush, Luu, & Posner, 2000; Haznedar et al., 1997; Luu & Posner, 2003); therefore, the variability across studies might reflect differential error processing for different types of tasks, or it may be indicative of state change or vigilance levels relative to task. Notably, animal studies demonstrating reactive or physical stress show the involvement of brainstem mechanisms while human studies on psychological stress or anxiety show activity in limbic and medial cortical regions (Figueiredo, Bodie, et al., 2003; Herman, Figueiredo, et al., 2003; Herman, Renda, & Bodie, 2003; Hermann et al., 2003). There is an intricate relationship between the AC and prefrontal mechanisms since it is extensively connected to the hippocampus (HC), hypothalamus, as well as brainstem (Herman, Flak, & Jankord, 2008; Jankord & Herman, 2008). As mentioned previously, with respect to the processing of psychological stress, the AC might play a role in individuals for whom a psychological stressor might represent both a social and physical threat.

It should be noted that data from animals and humans suggest a hierarchical integration of stress, where the influence of the PFC regions on the downstream regulators varies with region and nature of the stimulus (Herman, Figueiredo, et al., 2003) and possibly the nature of the regulatory and coping mechanisms of an individual. Specific EEG frequency domains in specific regions of the cortex may serve as accurate predictors of treatment response as well as provide specific characteristics of the disorder. Both qEEG and LORETA provide the opportunity to investigate generalized anxiety disorder as well as panic and social phobia in more detail and perhaps delineate state changes measured by neuroendocrine functions as they occur. This is an important direction for future studies.

3.3: Substance Use Disorders

Quantitative EEG and neuroimaging techniques have been used extensively to study substance related disorders (SUD). Since we can draw from large numbers of data, this review section will cover several lines of research. Compared to normal controls, alcohol-dependent patients consistently show an increase in absolute and relative beta power and a decrease in alpha and delta/theta power (Saletu, Anderer, Di Padova, Assandri, & Saletu-Zyhlarz, 2002).

It is suggested that lower frequency domains may be inhibitory with alpha activity being viewed as an expression of normal brain functioning and fast beta activities being viewed as excitatory. However, this view of the EEG frequency domains may be over simplistic. The low-voltage fast desynchronized patterns may be interpreted as an excitatory state of the central nervous system (CNS) (Saletu-Zyhlarz et al., 2004).

Alternatively, deficits in delta and theta frequencies may be indicative of limbic dysfunction, since delta and theta are the predominant limbic EEG rhythms in addition to their respective thalamo-cortical connections (Brazier, 1968). Of particular interest to SUD is recent data that demonstrate that alpha activity is shown to correlate significantly with white matter architecture (Valdes-Hernandez et al., 2010). However, we have to consider that parietal and occipital regions often show deficit in alpha/theta power and that neurofeedback training in these regions have produced positive results in treatment retention as well as personality measures (Peniston & Kulkosky, 1989). Bauer (Bauer,

2001; Bauer et al., 2001), and others (Winterer et al., 2003) indicated poorer prognoses for the patients exhibiting a more pronounced frontal fast activity.

The EEG features and LORETA maps of alcohol-dependent patients, which are significantly different from the EEG features and LORETA maps of normal controls and patients suffering from other mental disorders, may prove useful for both diagnostic and monitoring treatment efficacy purposes (Pollock, 1992; Saletu, Anderer, Saletu-Zyhlarz, & Pascual-Marqui, 2002). It is proposed that decreased power in slow bands in alcoholic patients may indicate brain atrophy and chronic brain damage, while increased beta band may relate to various factors, such as medication use, family history of alcoholism, and/ or hallucinations, suggesting a state of cortical hyperexcitability (Coutin-Churchman, Moreno, Anez, & Vergara, 2006).

Alternatively, the same slower frequencies are also implicated in cognitive and memory processes and play an important role in overall intelligence (Doppelmayr, Klimesch, Sauseng, et al., 2005; Jausovec & Jausovec, 2001; Polunina & Davydov, 2006; Tedrus, Fonseca, Tonelotto, Costa, & Chiodi, 2006; Thatcher, North, & Biver, 2005a, 2007; Thatcher et al., 2008); thus, this disagreement requires more clarity.

Abnormalities in resting EEG are often shown in individuals with a family history of alcoholism, such that these individuals were found to have reduced relative and absolute alpha power in occipital and frontal regions and increased relative beta in both regions compared to subjects with a negative family history of alcoholism. One important consideration for children of alcoholics is the stress and anxiety factor. In an extensive clinical work with these patients, all of them presented some form of stress, anxiety, or excessive fear in the developing years and as such, we might expect the changes in the EEG to be somewhat affected by the stress of living in an environment along with the difficulties associated with substance abuse (e.g., violence, emotional abuse, neglect). These results suggest that resting EEG alpha abnormalities are possibly linked to risk for alcoholism, although their etiological significance is unclear (Finn, Justus, Mazas, & Steinmetz, 1999).

Early studies on acute marijuana use showed increases in either posterior alpha power or decreases in the mean alpha amplitude as well as increases in alpha synchrony (Fink & Irwin, 1976; Struve, Straumanis, Patrick, & Price, 1989). Additionally, marijuana exposure produced an apparent dose-dependent rapid onset with increased relative power of alpha, decreased alpha frequency, and decreased relative beta power as measured by posterior scalp electrodes. Further studies demonstrate and replicate a significant association between chronic marijuana use and topographic qEEG patterns of persistent alpha in frontal regions as well as reductions in alpha mean frequency (Struve, Manno, Kemp, Patrick, & Manno, 2003; Struve, Patrick, Straumanis, Fitz-Gerald, & Manno, 1998). Chronic daily marijuana use, compared to non-use, is associated with distinct topographic qEEG features. Compared to nonusers, daily marijuana users show significant elevations of absolute and relative power with interhemispheric coherence increases in alpha activity over the bilateral frontal cortex. Similarly, nearly all other frequency bands were significantly elevated in marijuana users, although the amplitude increase was generalized and not frontally dominant. A widespread decrease in delta and beta activity was shown in cannabis users, with a particular effect over the frontal cortical regions. Recent data have demonstrated that heavy marijuana use may have deleterious effects on integrative processes due to the volume reduction and damage to white matter pathways with some preferential aspects in the corpus callosum (Arnone et al., 2008; Jacobus et al., 2009; Medina, Nagel, Park, McQueeny, & Tapert, 2007).

One of the more interesting qualities of SUD is that different substances produce many similar effects but dissimilar behaviors. Similar to alcohol, the effects of cocaine on human EEG exhibit an increase in activity in the beta frequency domain (Alper, 1999; Alper, Chabot, Kim, Prichep, & John, 1990; Prichep et al., 1999; Prichep, Kowalik, Alper, & de Jesus, 1995). In addition to these reported beta effects, some studies have reported an increase in delta activity and frontal alpha activity (Herning, Glover, Koeppl, Phillips, & London, 1994; Herning, Jones, Hooker, Mendelson, & Blackwell, 1985; Herning & King, 1996), while others have reported an increase in alpha that is associated with bursts of cocaine-induced euphoria (Lukas, Mendelson, Amass, & Benedikt, 1989). More recently, researchers have begun analyzing qEEG profiles of cocaine-dependent patients using the spectral power of each primary bandwidth over the different topographic cortical areas. The primary qEEG abnormalities associated with cocaine dependency were found over anterior cortical regions and were shown to correlate with the amount of prior cocaine use (Venneman et al., 2006). The qEEG has been used to characterize the effects of withdrawal in cocaine-dependent patients. Several studies reported predominant qEEG and long-term increases in alpha and beta bands inclusively with reduced activity in delta and theta bands during cocaine abstinence (Alper et al., 1990; Roemer, Cornwell, Dewart, Jackson, & Ercegovac, 1995).

Several conditions that have known neurophysiological aberrations, as described in earlier sections, are commonly associated with addictive disorders. The co-occurrence of alcohol and other SUD with other psychiatric disorders has been widely recognized. Co-occurrence of SUD and other psychiatric diagnoses (e.g., PTSD, antisocial personality disorder, ADHD, unipolar depression, etc.) is highly prevalent and important for developing successful, effective treatment strategies (Buckley, 2006; Drake & Wallach, 2000); Dual diagnosis. Part II. A look at old reliable and promising new approaches to the treatment of mental illness with substance abuse," 2003; Dual diagnosis: Part I. Mental illness and substance abuse can be a devastating combination, but help is increasingly available," (2003; Potvin et al., 2008; Smith, 2001; Wise, Cuffe, & Fischer, 2001). Persons with other co-occurring mental disorders and SUD have a more persistent illness course and are more resistant to the effects of treatment compared to those without a comorbid diagnosis (Araujo et al., 1996; Batson, Brown, Zaballero, Chu, & Alterman, 1993; Brown, Recupero, & Stout, 1995; Johnson, 1994; Neighbors, Kempton, & Forehand, 1992; Westermeyer, Kopka, & Nugent, 1997).

Depression occurs in approximately 30% of chronic alcoholics (Regier et al., 1990). Morphological differences between alcoholism and depression are reported to involve ventricular enlargement, which is more pronounced in depressive persons compared to alcoholics. Moreover, alcoholics tend to develop neuronal loss specific to the dorsolateral prefrontal cortex, suggesting that alcoholism, unlike depression, does not progress to other regions (Miguel-Hidalgo & Rajkowska, 2003). Hippocampal atrophy and decreased volume is reported in alcoholics but not in non-alcoholics (Bleich, Bandelow et al., 2003; Bleich, Sperling, et al., 2003; Bleich, Wilhelm, et al., 2003). Similarly, decreased volume in the prefrontal cortex is reported in crack-cocaine dependent men (Fein, Di Sclafani, & Meyerhoff, 2002).

Differences have been demonstrated between recovering substance abusers and controls in delta, theta, and upper alpha frequency domains in left dorsolateral prefrontal cortex (BA 9 and 6) and right occipital-parietal regions (BA 19) (Cannon, Baldwin, & Lubar, 2008). BA 19 is a region of the cortex considered a tertiary visual processing region in conjunction with BA 18. It is active during confrontation naming tasks (Abrahams et al., 2003), and its activity decreases when subjects make decisions about favorite brands of consumer goods (Deppe, Schwindt, Kugel, Plassmann, & Kenning, 2005). This occipital region has been shown active during unimodal visual motion stimulation (Deutschlander et al., 2002), stereodepth perceptions (Fortin, Ptito, Faubert, & Ptito, 2002), "theory of mind" tasks (Goel, Grafman, Sadato, & Hallett, 1995), and memory retrieval (Osipova et al., 2006).

Two points of interest regarding this region in relation to addiction are its connection with the hippocampus and right AC, which has been demonstrated in the study on the organization of pyramidal cells in the hippocampus (Casanova, Switala, & Trippe, 2007), and its involvement in perceptual processes involving the self and self in experience (Cannon, Baldwin, & Lubar, 2008). The regions in the left prefrontal cortex have been shown to be involved in working memory, disinhibition, and cognitive processes. Studies have shown that mental state considerations that explicitly reflect aspects of one's own mental state or attributions made about the mental states of others employ these dorsal anterior cingulate and dorsal medial prefrontal regions. Similarly, imaging studies targeting retrieval of personal or episodic memories involving verbal and nonverbal material have implicated the same prefrontal region. The deficits in left prefrontal and occipital regions may disrupt self-monitoring and self-evaluation processes that also involve limbic and brainstem fear centers (Cabeza, Dolcos, et al., 2003; Cabeza, Locantore, & Anderson, 2003; Cabeza & Nyberg, 2003; Cannon, Lubar, Sokhadze, & Baldwin, 2008; Frith, Friston, Liddle, & Frackowiak, 1991a; Frith, Friston, Liddle, & Frackowiak, 1991b; Liddell et al., 2005; Nyberg et al., 2003). Figure 31 shows regions of overlap in neuroimaging tasks involving self-relevance, autobiographical memory, reward, executive functions, drug related cues, emotional drug related cues, and other appetitive processes as well as numerous cognitive processes (Bush, 2008; Bush et al., 1999; Bush, Valera, & Seidman, 2005; Cannon, 2009; Cannon, Baldwin, & Lubar, 2008; Cannon et al., 2009; Fair et al., 2008; Fransson, 2006; Frei et al., 2001; Frith et al., 1991a; Goldstein, Alia-Klein, et al., 2007; Gusnard, Akbudak, Shulman, & Raichle, 2001; Gusnard et al., 2003; Herman & Cullinan, 1997; Lutz, Greischar, Perlman, & Davidson, 2009; Moriguchi et al., 2006; Panksepp & Northoff, 2009; Potenza, 2007; Uddin, Kaplan, Molnar-Szakacs, Zaidel, & Iacoboni, 2005; Vogeley & Fink, 2003). Importantly, the temporal lobe and insular cortices do not appear in the schematic, although both are vital to the processes listed. Similar activations exist in all disorders covered in this section, especially concerning reward (or reinforcement) mechanisms, default network, and emotional processing.

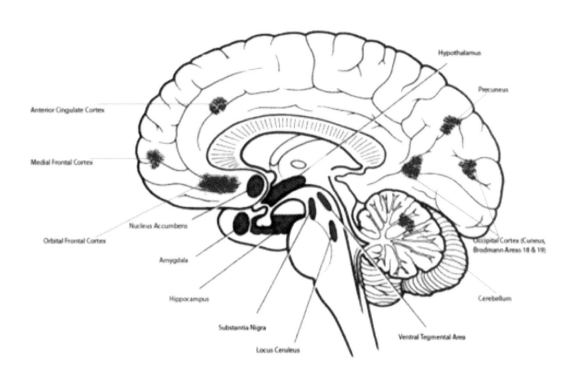

Figure 31: Schematic approximation of 2-D rendering of regional reward activations shown in fMRI experiments investigating drug related ques, emotional aspects of drug related words and self-referential processes.

In treatment settings, these depressed patients can present particular challenges to the clinicians, as they may not respond as well to the treatment as other patients, may have greater relapse, attrition, and readmission rates, and may manifest symptoms that are more severe, chronic, and refractory in nature (Sheehan, 1993).

Independent of other psychiatric comorbidity, ADHD alone significantly increases the risk for SUD (Biederman et al., 1995). Associated social and behavioral problems may make individuals with comorbid SUD and ADHD resistant to traditional cognitive, behavioral or therapeutic environment treatment paradigms (Wilens, Biederman, & Mick, 1998). In males aged 16 to 23 years, the presence of childhood ADHD and conduct disorder is associated with non-alcohol SUD (Gittelman, Mannuzza, Shenker, & Bonagura, 1985; Mannuzza, Fyer, et al., 1989; Mannuzza, Klein, Konig, & Giampino, 1989). In summary, childhood ADHD associated with conduct disorder in males is an antecedent of adult non-alcohol SUD and antisocial personality disorder (Wender, 1995). The incidence of ADHD in clinical SUD populations has been studied and may be as high as 50% for adults and adolescents (Downey, Stelson, Pomerleau, & Giordani, 1997; Horner & Scheibe, 1997). Adult residual ADHD is especially associated with cocaine abuse and other stimulant abuse (Levin & Kleber, 1995).

Furthermore, rates of PTSD occurring in persons primarily identified with, or in treatment for, substance abuse vary from 43% (Breslau, Davis, Andreski, & Peterson, 1991) up to 59% (Triffleman, Carroll, & Kellogg, 1999). Cocaine abusers were three times more likely to meet diagnostic criteria for PTSD compared to individuals without a SUD (Cottler, Compton, Mager, Spitznagel, & Janca, 1992). SUD is a very complex system of disorders, with a complimentary set of complex neural systems. Our lab will continue to examine recovering substance abusers using LORETA and functional MRI in order to examine the self and its neural mechanisms more intimately.

For a more indepth discussion of EEG parameters associated with substance use disorder see Sokhadze, Cannon & Trudeau (2008).

3.4: Attention Deficit/Hyperactivity Disorder

Recent reviews of Attention Deficit/Hyperactivity Disorder describe a consistent pattern of frontal dysfunction affecting closely related areas, such as dorsolateral prefrontal cortex, anterior cingulate, ventrolateral prefrontal cortex, parietal cortex, and striatal and cerebellar regions (Bush, 2008; Bush et al., 1999; Bush & Shin, 2006; Bush et al., 2008; Bush et al., 2005). Similarly, structural magnetic resonance imaging (MRI) and EEG studies of ADHD report that reductions in frontal and caudate nuclei volume are the most frequently detected abnormalities. qEEG studies have demonstrated consistent differences between control and ADHD children, with ADHD children showing increased frontal theta activity, increased posterior delta activity, and decreased alpha and beta activity (Willis & Weiler, 2005). A classification model was based on theta/beta power ratios and reported classification rates of ADHD and control subjects reaching 86% sensitivity and 98% specificity (Monastra, 2005, 2008; Monastra, Lubar, & Linden, 2001; Monastra et al., 1999; Monastra et al., 2005; Monastra, Monastra, & George, 2002). Recent data support these findings with a similarly high classification rate of ADHD detection in a diverse clinical sample and by showing that both rating scales and EEG are both sensitive markers, whereas only EEG is specific (Quintana, Snyder, Purnell, Aponte, & Sita, 2007).

Studies have frequently conducted functional neuroimaging investigations of brain activation patterns in ADHD in response to cognitively demanding tasks. These studies have shown that differences in cognitive control between subjects with and without ADHD are associated with differences in brain activation patterns (Bush et al., 1999; Bush et al., 2002; Durston, 2003; Durston et al., 2003; Rubia, 2002; Rubia et al., 2001; Rubia, Smith, Taylor, & Brammer, 2007). In particular, reduced activation in prefrontal areas as well as linked decreases in the recruitment of striatal regions during paradigms that require subjects to suppress (or self-regulate) responses as part of the task, such as in the go/no-go or Stroop paradigms (Bush et al., 1999; Rubia, 2002; Zang et al., 2005). This research paradigm has demonstrated the anterior cingulate gyrus to be less responsive in ADHD populations compared to controls and has led to the suggestion that these functional regional deficits are central to ADHD (Bush et al., 2005).

Neuroimaging studies have also investigated behavioral control, attention, mental rotation, and employed tasks, and their association with motivated behavior, such as a reward anticipation task (Konrad, Neufang, Hanisch, Fink, & Herpertz-Dahlmann, 2006;

Scheres, Milham, Knutson, & Castellanos, 2007; Silk et al., 2005). The results show deficits in striatal and prefrontal activation as well as changes in activation in parietal areas. The general findings emphasize the importance of fronto-striatal networks in ADHD. Although there is no definitive physiological model of ADHD, further evidence for fronto-striatal impairment in ADHD comes from the research on stimulant medications as well as animal models of hyperactivity that implicate dopamine pathways associated with these regions (Gainetdinov et al., 1999).

More recently, neural regions involved in the reward system have been investigated. Data indicated differences between ADHD adults and controls in regions containing the dopamine D2/D3 receptor and the dopamine transporter in the left ventral striatum (including accumbens and ventral caudate), left midbrain, and left hypothalamus (Volkow et al., 2009). Similar findings on reward mechanisms, previously reported in adolescents and adults with ADHD, have shown that adults with ADHD showed less activity in ventral striatum to immediately available rewards (Scheres, Lee, & Sumiya, 2008; Strohle et al., 2008). However, the ADHD sample also differed from controls such that increased activity to delayed rewards occurred in dorsal striatal regions. The delay aversion theory of ADHD suggests that delayed rewards should be associated with negative emotional responses, which would be expected to involve the amygdala. The results further indicate a significantly lesser degree of activation in the amygdala to immediate rewards and increased activity in the amygdala to delayed rewards in the ADHD sample. Additionally, hyperactivity/ impulsivity symptom severity scales were significantly and positively associated with BOLD levels in both dorsal caudate and amygdala (Sonuga-Barke, Taylor, & Heptinstall, 1992; Sonuga-Barke, Taylor, Sembi, & Smith, 1992).

The first functional imaging study of ADHD using PET in adults reported decreased glucose metabolism in superior frontal, premotor, and cingulate cortices among ADHD adults compared to controls (Zametkin et al., 1990). Additional research showed that during a working memory task, rCBF activation differences between controls and ADHD patients were found in frontal and temporal regions (Schweitzer et al., 2000). Structural MRI data indicated reduced left orbitofrontal cortex volumes in ADHD adults relative to control subjects (Hesslinger et al., 2002). Structural imaging data in children with ADHD showed anomalous findings in the basal ganglia, cerebellum, and corpus callosum (Seidman, Valera, & Bush, 2004). Although the frontal lobes are the most investigated region in ADHD, consistent findings show volume reductions in the cerebellum, caudate, and corpus callosum (Castellanos, 2001; Castellanos et al., 2003; Castellanos & Tannock, 2002).

The neurological substrates of ADHD remain ambiguous. It has been proposed that ADHD involves abnormalities in an "attention system" of the brain comprising anterior frontostriatal components and posterior parietal cortex (Pardo, Fox, & Raichle, 1991; Posner, 1994; Posner & Dehaene, 1994), particularly in the right hemisphere. Recent data suggest a distributed bilateral anterior-posterior executive attention network in normal populations, with emphasis on right fronto-parietal involvement in all EEG frequency domains (Cannon et al., 2009).

People with ADHD have been shown to have a reduction in the total volume of the brain, with both white and grey matter showing significant reductions compared to control. A preliminary voxel-based study of ADHD reported predominantly right hemispheric grey matter deficits in basal ganglia, superior frontal gyrus, and posterior cingulate (Overmeyer et al., 2001). A recent comprehensive review of structural imaging studies on ADHD noted that many previous studies have been conducted with fewer than 20 patients. Additionally, the review implicated language, ethnicity, gender, and environmental influences in overall brain differences (Seidman, Valera, & Makris, 2005).

MRI data have also demonstrated important volume reductions in dorsolateral prefrontal and anterior cingulate cortices in adults with ADHD (Seidman et al., 2006). These regions were shown to be functionally correlated in the maintenance of executive attention in conjunction with right parietal and posterior cingulate cortices (Cannon et al., 2009). In a voxel based study on regional grey and white matter volumes in 28 male children with ADHD, grey matter volume deficits were more extensive in the right hemisphere, especially in the prefrontal lobe (BA9, BA10), globus pallidus, and medial parietal cortex (BA7) in ADHD children compared to controls (McAlonan et al., 2007). Similarly, reduced grey matter volume was also measured in the left inferior parietal lobe and superior occipital gyrus.

The authors also reported smaller white matter volume in ADHD children that was distributed bilaterally in frontal, temporal, and parietal lobes. The main findings of this study were that, compared to controls, children with ADHD had localized grey matter deficits in predominantly right-sided fronto-parietal brain networks as well as significant volume reduction in associated white matter tracts but no significant differences in whole brain volume or in total volume of grey or white brain matter or CSF (McAlonan et al., 2007).

Interestingly the authors underlined the important role of the cerebellum in the pathogenesis of ADHD, which is in line with the conceptualization that the cerebellum is involved in higher order cognition, including executive function, through intimate reciprocal connections with frontostriatal regions (Leiner, Leiner, & Dow, 1989; McAlonan et al., 2007; Middleton & Strick, 1994).

The default mode network (DMN) in the human brain is an area of concentrated study. It is discussed in more detail later in this text. However, the DMN, which is specific to ADHD, is important due to its functional components comprising medial (medial prefrontal cortex, posterior cingulate/precuneus) and lateral (posterior parietal) brain regions that routinely exhibit coherent decreases in activity during attention-demanding cognitive tasks (Raichle et al., 2001). It has also been noted that attentional lapses have been found to occur shortly after periods of decreased deactivation of posterior DMN regions (Weissman, Roberts, Visscher, & Woldorff, 2006).

ADHD is a diverse developmental condition with various potential loci of neural dysfunction. Recent data indicate decreased functional connectivity between the precuneus and other DMN regions in adults with ADHD (Castellanos et al., 2008), with additional data indicating decreased DMN network homogeneity in the precuneus in ADHD compared to controls (Castellanos et al., 2008).

The functional connectivity finding is a common finding of studies using qEEG and LORETA in clinical samples of children and adults with ADHD, as shown in the provided clinical samples. The precuneus is a prominent node in the DMN that has been given an increased attention in the ADHD neuroimaging literature. Research has shown reductions in grey matter volume in the precuneus in ADHD samples (Carmona et al., 2005; Overmeyer et al., 2001). The precuneus has been shown to play an important role in cognitive and self-relevant processing (Enzi, de Greck, Prosch, Tempelmann, & Northoff, 2009; Northoff, 2005; Northoff & Bermpohl, 2004; Northoff et al., 2006; Northoff et al., 2009). It may also play an important function in affect and self-regulatory functions given its widespread connectivity with anterior cingulate, lateral prefrontal, inferior and superior parietal lobes, and sub-cortical connections, including the thalamus, striatum, and brainstem regions (Cavanna & Trimble, 2006).

Importantly, all regions in the default network can be monitored with qEEG and LORETA methods (Cannon, 2009; Cannon et al., 2009). Additionally, LORETA neurofeedback can be implemented in DMN regions including the anterior cingulate and precuneus (Cannon et al., 2009; Cannon et al., 2007; Cannon et al., 2008; Cannon,

Baldwin, & Lubar, 2009). Important data also indicate that the fronto-insular cortex plays an important role in the transition between executive attention and default network activity (Sridharan, Levitin, & Menon, 2008). Figure 32 shows the results of LORETA neurofeedback training of 14-18 Hz (low-beta) power in the cognitive division of the AC in monozygotic twins with ADHD.

Figure 33 shows the active training rounds for the twins compared to a sample of eight controls that completed the same training. Compared to dorsolateral prefrontal and parietal activations in controls, especially concerning DMN regions, the AC training in these twins shows the largest increase in bilateral insula (Cannon et al., 2009; Cannon et al., 2007).

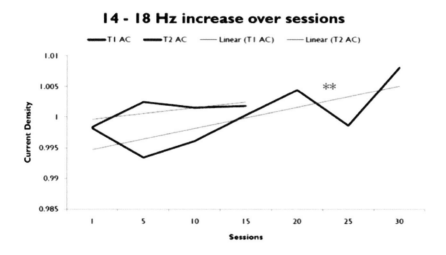

Figure 32: Learning curve for monozygotic twins concordant with ADHD (inattentive type) for LNFB in the left dorsal anterior cingulate.

Importantly, in ADHD but not in controls, the left precuneus region has been shown to produce the largest effect across all relative frequency domains (BA 19). Both twins were able to increase current source density in the AC over sessions, as shown in Figure 33 (next page), although twin 2 dropped out after 15 sessions twin 1 showed a significant

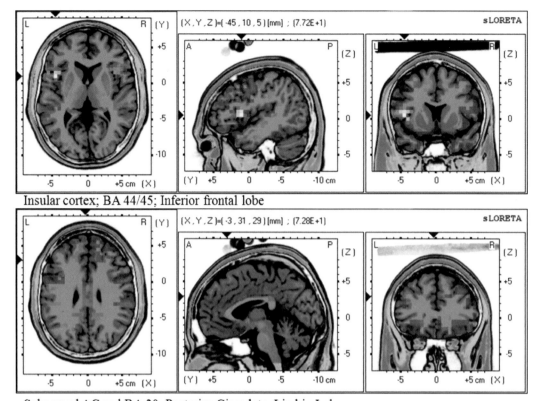

Insular cortex; BA 44/45; Inferior frontal lobe

Subgenual AC and BA 30; Posterior Cingulate; Limbic Lobe

Figure 33: Horizontal slices through the brain of twins during the active LNFB training protocols. Figure 33. These images are statistical comparisons of the training rounds (increasing 14 - 18 Hz activity) in the dorsal anterior cingulate gyrus. While the cingulate did show learning effects, as indicated in figure 32, the greatest increase in network connectivity occurred in the bilateral insular cortex, with higher levels shown in the right insula. This is important since this region is possibly involved in a moderation role over the default network.

learning trend over sessions. However, connectivity between the AC and other regions in a network of executive attention did not follow the same pattern in controls (Cannon et al., 2009). Other regions of significant increase shown in Figure 33 are parahippocampal gyri, BA 37, 6, 36, and 35 respectively. Twin 1 showed a significant improvement in learning, as shown in Figure 32.

Recent research (Silk et al., 2005; Vance et al., 2007) utilizing diffusion tensor imaging has shown dysfunction of a larger, more extensive attentional, cognitive, and visuospatial network that involves frontal, striatal, and parietal areas. The authors indicated that this network is of fundamental importance for attentional and cognitive control (Mesulam, 1990). The important clusters of significance were located in the white-matter underlying right occipito-parietal cortex, left inferior frontal cortex/striatum, and left inferior temporal regions. Regions approaching significance were also reported in white-matter underlying right inferior parietal and left inferior frontal regions (Silk, Vance, Rinehart, Bradshaw, & Cunnington, 2009).

Attention deficit hyperactivity disorder (ADHD) is a developmental psychiatric disorder affecting approximately 4% of school-age children, of whom 30% to 65% continue to exhibit symptoms into adulthood (Faraone, Biederman, & Mick, 2006). Individuals with ADHD tend to suffer reduced educational outcomes and an increased incidence of comorbid psychiatric syndromes, including substance abuse, antisocial behavior, anxiety, and depression (Spencer, Biederman, & Mick, 2007). The etiology of ADHD and exact neurological substrates are unknown, additionally the interactions between genetics and environmental influences are still unclear. However, there appears to be significant network dysfunctions involved in ADHD across studies. The DMN, insular cortices, frontal lobes, basal ganglia, and cerebellum are foci of interest, with a more recent focus on the precuneus and parietal lobes and their interactions with anterior cingulate (Castellanos, 2001; Castellanos & Acosta, 2002; Castellanos, Glaser, & Gerhardt, 2006; Castellanos et al., 2008).

Recent reviews of the available ADHD treatments have proposed that cognitive behavioral methods are inadequate (Toplak, Connors, Shuster, Knezevic, & Parks, 2008) while neurofeedback offers a more efficacious and specific treatment option (Arns, de Ridder, Strehl, Breteler, & Coenen, 2009). ADHD is treated predominantly with stimulant medications, such as methylphenidate or amphetamine, which primarily release and prevent the reuptake of catecholamines (dopamine and noradrenaline) (Arnsten, 2006).

These stimulant medications have been demonstrated to bring about a transitory reduction in ADHD symptoms in medication responsive patients and as such have led to the focus on dopaminergic and noradrenergic pathways in the neurobiology of ADHD (O'Gorman et al., 2008). As our understanding of the intrinsic network properties of the brain increases, so does our need to understand the dynamics of the EEG within and between these networks. qEEG and LORETA may play an important role in this discovery process.

3.5: Clinical Examples

Figure 34, page 92, shows LORETA images for various clinical cases. The patients' ages and syndromes are noted below the images. The images are horizontal, sagittal, and coronal views of the brain that show the x, y, and z coordinates as well as the TF (or frequency domains in 1 Hz increments), all in the alpha frequency domain.

The blue in the image indicates a decreased current source density (CSD) as compared to the Life-span Database (Thatcher, Biver, & North, 2003) with Neuroguide (Applied Neuroscience Laboratories), which permits a comparison of the estimated intracerebral current density distribution with LORETA (Thatcher, North, & Biver, 2005b, 2005c). As noted in earlier chapters, the red indicates regions of significantly increased CSD, while the blue indicates regions of significantly decreased CSD as compared to the Life-span Database. The Life-span Database allows for a comparison to a normative sample without the collection of a local control group.

Thus, EEG is the only neuroimaging technique that allows statistical comparison of individual recordings with age-matched or age-regressed life-span normative databases (Hughes & John, 1999; John et al., 1988; Thatcher et al., 2005b, 2005c). The recordings in Figure 34, obtained with the Deymed Truscan EEG acquisition system with 19 leads (10/20 system), linked ear reference. The EEG was artifacted and the selected segments for analysis showed test-retest alpha of >.90 for all patients. The total time for the analyzed EEG was > 1.30 minutes. These analyses were all conducted in the eyes-opened attentive-resting state.

As mentioned earlier in the text, alpha activity may have a potential white-matter function (Valdes-Hernandez et al., 2010) as opposed to the traditional pacemaker function proposed in earlier data (Garoutte & Aird, 1958; Rosen & Robinson, 1990). Additionally, alpha appears to play a substantial role in perceptual mechanisms related to negative or positive self-perception processes in recovering substance abusers and normal controls (Cannon, 2009; Cannon, Baldwin, & Lubar, 2008), as well as in attention, cognitive and memory processes, and ADHD (Angelakis, Lubar, & Stathopoulou, 2004; Angelakis, Lubar, Stathopoulou, et al., 2004; Angelakis et al., 2007; Swartwood, Swartwood, Lubar, & Timmermann, 2003; Timmermann, Lubar, Rasey, & Frederick, 1999). Interestingly, similar deficits in the alpha frequency domain are noted across age, gender, and psychiatric syndromes. Of course, other anomalies are also noted in other frequency domains of each specific disorder; however, considering frequency interactions and effects between patients, the alpha deficits represent a novel research direction. Based on this deficit pattern, we have implemented a neurofeedback protocol, submitted for publication in 2011, to address the alpha deficit and concomitant increases or decreases in other frequency domains. Importantly, from a simple observation standpoint, alpha does appear to be important foci for the development of neurofeedback protocols addressing parietal-precuneus regions of interest.

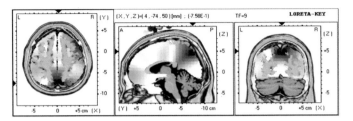

A: (9 year old boy) Impulsivity | Transient facial tics | Explosive anger outbursts

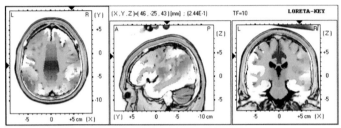

B: (9 year old boy) Asperger's syndrome

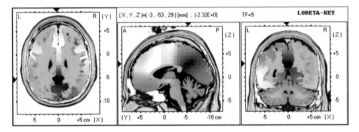

C: (9 year old boy) Lesion in posterior cingulate/corpus collosum

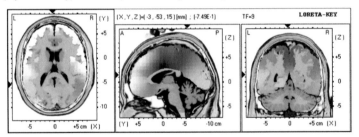

D: (37 year old female) Anxiety/Depression

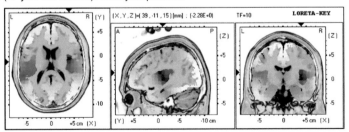

E: (12 year old girl) ADHD

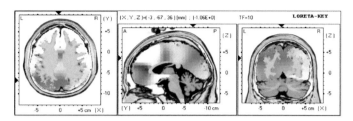

F: (49 year old female) Anxiety/Panic/Depression

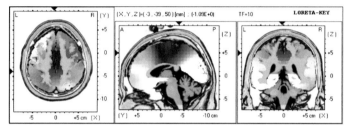

:G: (23 year old male) SUD - after a night of IV cocaine use

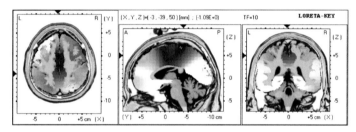

H: (10 year old boy) ADHD

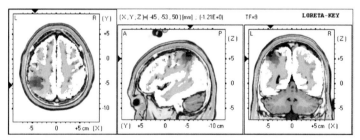

I: (25 year old male) SUD in remission/comorbid ADHD since age 6

Figure 34-A-I: LORETA maps compared to Lifespan database. Parietal deficits in alpha are prevalent across age, gender and disorder, indicating variable hemispheric effects.

3.6: Monitoring Treatment Effects

Treatment outcomes, evidence based methods, and monitoring treatment efficacy are important considerations for qEEG and LORETA. Research into the possible neural effects of psychotherapy as efficacy and outcome measures has experienced a rather slow development. The noninvasive functional brain imaging techniques can now reliably detect training and learning related changes in brain activation patterns in healthy volunteers, and this should now be possible in those affected by mental disorders. Recent studies on the default network, resting state networks, and functional connectivity techniques afford the opportunity to study basic brain mechanisms as well as treatment response, treatment efficacy, and the neural changes (or no changes) that occur as a result of the therapeutic process.

These recent developments offer the potential to select a region of interest *a priori* to monitor in post treatment analysis. Further analytic techniques can then be employed to simply observe change and provide important information relative to the subjective experience or state change of the patient. Such an approach would not only benefit basic research on the mechanisms of action of psychotherapy, but would also increase our understanding of differences and commonalities between psycho- and pharmacotherapy. Several neuroimaging studies have investigated Cognitive Behavior Therapy and pharmacotherapy. The major findings in obsessive-compulsive disorder showed increased activity in the right caudate in symptom provocation across imaging modalities (Breiter et al., 1996; Rauch et al., 1994). The effects of cognitive behavioral therapy (CBT) in OCD on resting state glucose metabolism or blood flow have thus far reported a decrease in right caudate activity in treatment responders (Baxter et al., 1992; Schwartz, Stoessel, Baxter, Martin, & Phelps, 1996). This decrease in caudate activity correlated with clinical improvement in one study while showing no difference in caudate activity between CBT and treatment with the selective serotonin reuptake inhibitor (SSRI) fluoxetine. Two studies reported a correlation between caudate, OFC, and thalamus activity before the treatment, conforming to current pathophysiological models of OCD (Brody et al., 1998; Saxena, Brody, Schwartz, & Baxter, 1998; Schwartz, 1998).

Further investigation of the effects of behavioral interventions and the associated qEEG and LORETA sources would enhance our knowledge base and provide invaluable information about the possible frequency specific interactions involved in these pathologies. Similar studies of patients with social phobia have also shown increased activity in the amygdala. This increased activity was shown to continue after symptom provocation (Birbaumer et al., 1998; Furmark et al., 2002). Because of successful treatment, either with CBT or citalopram, activation of amygdala and hippocampus was reduced in a public speaking task. Again, it is interesting to observe that the pharmacological and psychological interventions seem to have modulated the same brain areas, in this case, parts of the limbic system. CBT and SSRI appear to produce similar effects on metabolic patterns, specifically by influencing the reduction in the activity of fronto-striatothalamic circuits. Many studies on resting state blood flow or metabolism reported normalization of an anterior prefrontal hypoperfusion after the remission of depression symptoms (Mayberg et al., 2002; Navarro et al., 2002). Decreases and normalizations have also been shown in lateral prefrontal regions in the successful treatment of depression (Goldapple et al., 2004; Seminowicz et al., 2004). More interestingly, LORETA neurofeedback techniques have been employed to address the limbic power abnormalities in the remission of depressive symptoms (Paquette, Beauregard, & Beaulieu-Prevost, 2009). These normalization effects are also shown in qEEG studies investigating the effects of medication on coherence and power anomalies in depression (Hughes & John, 1999). Treatment effects have also been evaluated in specific phobias, with patients showing a higher degree of activity in visual association areas for aversive rather than neutral sequences, which is similar to the pattern observed in the healthy controls. Again, CBT appears to have influenced a normalization of cortical processing specific to the spider sequences. Patients showed higher activation in the ACC and insula bilaterally when pretreatment fMRI was compared to healthy controls. This pattern of increased activation was present in the second measurement in the waiting list group, but was not present in the group treated with CBT. This reduction of ACC and insula activity might reflect the attenuation or modulation of the affective response to spiders after successful treatment (Paquette et al., 2003; Straube, Glauer, Dilger, Mentzel, & Miltner, 2006).

At present, the available evidence suggests that any model that relies on global frontal hypometabolism to explain symptoms of depression and its reversal to account for treatment effects would be oversimplifying the complex nature of cortico-cortical and subcortical interactions in affective and other psychological disorders. Alternatively, our knowledge base of functional connectivity and neural hubs and nodes within the brain during baseline and active tasks offers an encouraging direction for the use of EEG localization techniques in monitoring state specific processes (Cannon, Thatcher, Lubar, & Baldwin, 2009; Cannon, 2009) for monitoring treatment effects. It is also important to consider that the average psychotherapy or neurofeedback patient will not be able to afford an fMRI or PET scan to determine treatment effectiveness; thus, the non-invasive and inexpensive properties of EEG and LORETA make it an ideal technique for such methods.

3.7: Clinical Examples and qEEG/LORETA-Guided Neurofeedback

Respective training programs emphasize that psychological and psychiatric treatment paradigms follow a scientist-practitioner-research model, using the identification of specific parameters (symptoms) associated with specific conditions to rule out other possible solutions. In a statistical sense, this is a step-wise reduction of factors to determine the best fit to the specific symptoms for the patient in order to determine the best fitting treatment paradigm. Neurotherapeutic (neurotherapy or neurofeedback) techniques introduce the potential to integrate the human brain in its rightful place at the forefront of the equation for assessing functional behavior and as such, provide a very powerful paradigm to monitor changes and understand basic behavioral mechanisms at their source. Neurotherapy may provide specific positive changes as a standalone procedure or as an adjunct or concordant procedure with other established behavioral, cognitive, or pharmacotherapy techniques. In the next few pages, I will review some clinical examples of the effects of qEEG guided neurofeedback training and cases in which the qEEG/ LORETA information complimented structural MRI and neuropsychological data.

In thinking about the empirical need for qEEG/LORETA guided neurofeedback, one prevalent notion indicates that a starting point must be established to have an ending point. In simplest terms, an outcome must be established in order to measure efficacy. As an example, I will discuss a case of traumatic brain injury with the qEEG and LORETA maps over a course of NF therapy. The first data discussed is from a 37-year-old, Caucasian male with traumatic brain injury (TBI) that resulted from an automobile accident. Neurofeedback was implemented nearly 10 years post trauma due to his desire to address memory problems, severe grand-mal seizures, prominent tremors, and difficulty in communicating and self-regulating. Figure 35 shows the pre-training eyes-closed baseline.

Tremors were quite profound extending to upper extremities; thus, his caregiver was asked to help stabilize body movements to obtain the recording. Substantial high amplitude slow activity and increased fast activity in parieto-occipital regions were noted. Figure 36 shows the EEG sources as contrasted with age similar controls in the lifespan database.

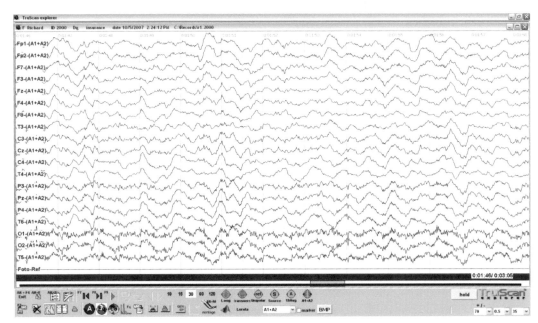

Figure 35: Pre NF training ECB. 6 seconds of EEG, note the high amplitude slow wave activity and faster frequencies in the occipital regions. Tremors were present and caregiver had to aid in helping the patient remain for the recordings.

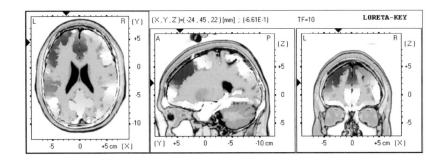

Figure 36: Pre ECB LORETA CSD showing severe deficits of alpha in frontal regions and contra-lateral parieto-occipital regions. He also showed extreme deficits in slower frequencies in frontal regions, with the exception of increased delta in left fronto-temporal regions.

There are significant deficits in left prefrontal, anterior cingulate and parieto-temporal regions. Given the degree of language, memory, and self-regulatory functions as well as seizure activity, the sources of deficit were considered to be highly related to his particular symptoms. Figure 37 shows the post training eyes-closed baseline (ECB) traces after 60 sessions of alpha training (amplitude) in left parietal-occipital region (between O1 and P3).

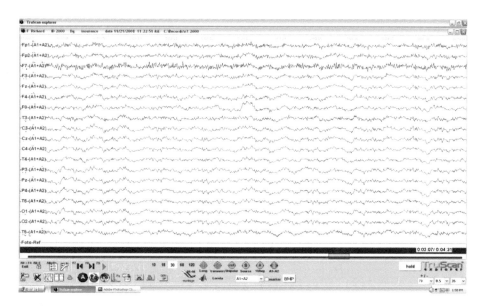

Figure 37: ECB recording at session 60. The high amplitude slow activity has subsided substantially. In combination with medications, the seizures have reduced significantly, language has markedly improved, and tremors have diminished; however, working memory has improved only moderately.

There was a significant reduction in higher amplitude slow activity and tremors. This location was selected according to the empirical data supporting the role of left parieto-occipital regions in language, memory, and self-regulatory processes. Delta and low-theta (1 - 5 Hz) activity was inhibited at T3/F3. Figure 38 shows the differences between pre and post NF training measures. The most notable increase was at BA 31 posterior cingulate with additional significant increases in frontal and parietal regions.

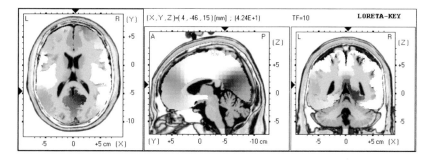

Figure 38: Difference between pre ECB and session 60 ECB. Significant increases were noted in frontal, parieto-occipital regions with the largest increase at BA 31 posterior cingulate, shown in the mid-alpha frequency (10 Hz).

Figure 39 shows the pre training eyes-opened baseline (EOB). The tremors were more intense in the EOB with notably high amplitude slow activity as well as increased faster frequencies in parieto-occipital regions.

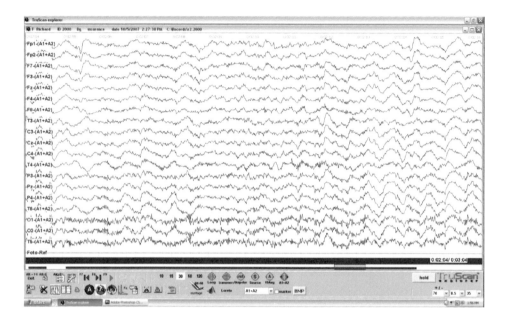

Figure 39: Pre EOB recording with high amplitude low frequencies and asynchronous patterns throughout the EEG. Excessive high frequency activity is shown in parieto-occipital regions.

Figure 40 shows the EEG sources for EOB as contrasted with age similar adults in the lifespan database. Similar to the ECB, there are significant deficits in frontal, anterior cingulate, and parieto-temporal cortices. Importantly, there is agreement between ECB and EOB recordings in the regions of deficit or excess activity.

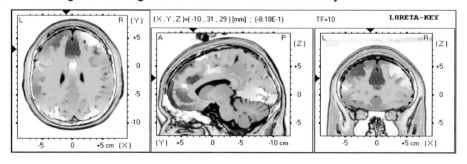

Figure 40: LORETA CSD for pre training EOB. Deficits in mid alpha are shown in left prefrontal and anterior cingulate gyrus.

Figure 41 shows the post EOB EEG traces at 60 sessions. There is a dramatic difference between the records that could also be observed in behavior, such that speech and communication were clearer, tremors and seizures were significantly reduced, and interpersonal behavior was improved.

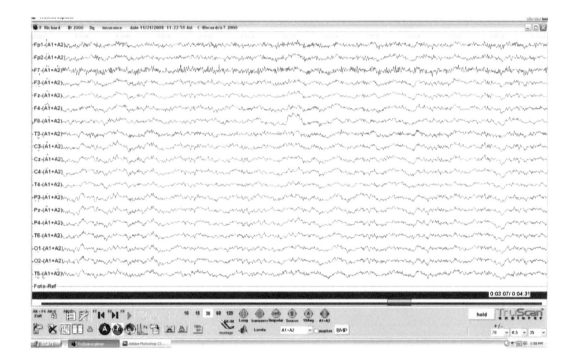

Figure 41: EOB baseline at session 60. The high amplitude activity has diminished significantly as did the higher frequencies in parieto-occipital leads.

Figure 42 shows the contrast between EOB at time 60 versus pre. The primary regional increase is shown in the posterior-temporal regions in the parahippocampal gyrus, precuneus, posterior cingulate and occipital cortex. Again, improvements in these regions potentially reflect the improvements in symptoms.

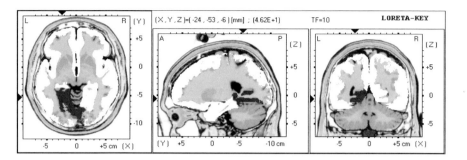

Figure 42: Significant differences between pre EOB and session 60 EOB recordings in the 10Hz alpha frequency range are noted. The specific areas that show increase are BA 19/18, 30, and 32 - scaling does not show frontal increases, as they were much lower than posterior regions.

This is but one example of how changes in the EEG are monitored with qEEG and LORETA to demonstrate the efficacy of NF as well as other treatment paradigms. Moreover, the presented data stress the importance of an interdisciplinary approach to specific syndromes. Certainly, without medications and their effects specifically on seizure activity, the NF paradigm may not have been as effective. Notably, the memory issues are the focus of an updated paradigm to influence low-beta power at F3 and inhibit slower frequencies.

This patient's results still show dramatic deficits compared to the database while showing significant improvements compared to pre NF. His overall functioning has improved in the area of motor control, tremor reduction, seizure reduction, and speech production and communication. Thus, the combinations of NF and medications have made a substantial effect on his global functioning.

The next clinical case report is for a 9-year-old, left-handed Caucasian with a medical history that includes perinatal subarachnoid hemorrhage and associated seizures. Seizures were adequately addressed with anticonvulsants. Parental report indicated that patient suffered paresis on the right side of his body that was present at time of discharge from hospital. However, with recommendations for physical therapy, his prognosis for recovery at 13-months was good, as EEG and CT findings did not indicate any focal abnormalities. His standing diagnoses at time of evaluation were Central Auditory Processing Disorder (CAPD) and Abnormal Auditory Processing, unspecified.

This was an important case study simply because years of testing by the education system and other clinicians did not produce any definitive diagnoses for the patient. The cumulative results of testing, until the time of our evaluation, revealed that primary deficits in neurocognitive functions were attributable to CAPD or other Auditory Processing Disorders. The summaries and disagreements between several test results may be the consequence of non-specific neuropsychological testing. In short, educational assessment may not be sensitive to specific neurocognitive dysfunctions and the important correlative structure between cognitive domains. Therefore, a brief neuropsychological screening using portions of the Reitan Battery for the Neuropsychological Evaluation of Children was employed. Additionally, simple tests of working memory, visual-spatial, language functions including category naming (verbal fluency), auditory and visual attention, and arithmetic were also performed.

Specifically, the patient was given several working memory tasks, including recall of numbers, letters, and words. When asked to recall the presented items, he was able to retain on average one of the three presented items, regardless of format. He was given 6 arithmetic problems with simple addition and subtraction using symbols, numbers, and word problems. He was able to complete the number problems rapidly and correctly. Symbols and word problems were the most difficult for him, and he made the most errors on these tasks. He was given a clock drawing and complex figure copying tasks. The clock was drawn semi-circular with numbers irregularly spaced, and the clock hands were not drawn and placed at the correct time (3:45). Notably, he did point at the clock, identifying the correct location of the clock hands. Specific parts of the complex figure were crude (diamond and triangle) but correctly drawn; however, integrating the gestalt was not achieved. Verbal fluency was assessed with category (animal) naming. The patient was asked to name as many animals as he could within one-minute. The patient could name only 8 in the allotted time. Reading was assessed on several occasions with a predominant pattern of slow, deliberate attempts to comply with the task. This pattern of reading was also present when reading a book that he had read on numerous occasions with his father at home. He was able to write out his name and the alphabet. He could recall and write out the 12-months of the year using only abbreviations. He was oriented to the month and date but did not know the year. He was able to recall his birthday and age. His scores on the integrative visual and auditory continuous performance tasks (IVA+Plus) indicated extreme deficits in both auditory and visual comprehension, mild deficits in sensory motor processes and scores within normal persistence limits in both auditory and visual domains. Additionally, an extreme number of hyperactive events were indicated. In sum, the child was extremely cooperative and effortful in attempts to comply with instructions. Parents did not report odd or aggressive behaviors.

Four-minute eyes-closed and eyes-opened resting baseline recordings were obtained with the Deymed Truscan EEG acquisition system with 19-leads (10/20 system) and linked-ear reference. The EEG was artifacted using Neuroguide (Applied Neuroscience laboratories) and the selected segments for analysis showed test-retest coefficient of >.90 between all segments. The total time for the analyzed EEG for EOB and ECB recordings was > 1.30 minutes. The EOB and ECB samples were compared with age-matched individuals from the life-span EEG normative database. The LORETA images were obtained and analyzed nearly 45 days prior to the MRI scans.

The Magnetic Resonance Imaging (MRI) Brain & Stem without contrast scans were conducted with a Siemens 1.5 T Avanto scanner (Siemens Medical Solutions, Erlangen, Germany) located in the Department of Radiology at the University of Tennessee Medical Center. Head restraint with headphones and cushions was used to immobilize the subject to minimize movement artifacts and attenuate echo noise. Axial T2-weighted images were obtained with the following parameters: Spin Echo (Se)=10/11, Repetition Time (TR)= 3400.0, Echo Time (TE)= 99.9, and Dynamic Field of View (DFOV)= 20.0 x 20.0 cm. Coronal T2-weighted images were obtained with Se=: 11/11, TR= 3516.7, TE= 88.1, and DFOV= 18.0 x 18.0 cm. Sagittal T1-weighted images were obtained with SE= 8/11, TE= 0, TR= 650.0, TE= 14.0, and DFOV= 22.0x 22.0 cm. The images were degraded due to motion artifacts. A board certified neuroradiologist and a board certified neurologist clinically evaluated the MRI scans.

The results of the MRI/LORETA procedures are shown in the figures below. On the left side of each figure is the MRI image and on the right is the LORETA image in a specific 1 Hz frequency interval. Figure 43 shows an axial T2-weighted image showing multifocal Encephalomalacia with surrounding gliosis most pronounced in the frontal lobes near the anterior and middle cerebral artery watershed distributions. The basal ganglia and brain stem are intact, except for a minimal disturbance in the anterior portion of the left caudate. The encephalomalacic changes are also seen in parietal regions with more pronounced effects in the left hemisphere that extend to the perisylvian region. The left hemisphere is shown in the right of the MRI image. The corresponding LORETA image is for the alpha frequency (10 Hz). The areas in red indicate z-scores with significant increased current source density, while the areas in blue indicate z-scores with significant decreased current source density compared to the database. The maximum region of decreased current source density in the mid-alpha range of 10Hz is shown at posterior cingulate/precuneus (x = -10, y = -53, z = 29) with a z-score of -2.08. Similar z scores were observed for the inferior parietal lobes (BA 40), with higher z-scores in the left hemisphere. This pattern is similar for all frequencies, with the exception of mid beta in the right hemisphere. Higher deficits in the beta frequency domain extend to the left insula and auditory processing regions.

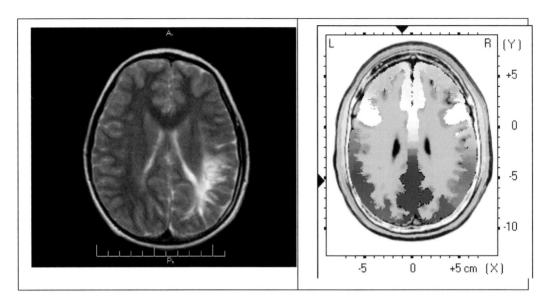

Figure 43: The left image shows a T2-weighted axial image of 9-year-old male showing multifocal areas of Encephalomalacia (EPm). EPm changes with surrounding gliosis are most pronounced in the frontal lobes near the ACA/MAC watershed distributions and are also present in both parietal lobes with left (in the right of the image) showing more pronounced infarcts near the perisylvian region. There is also disproportionate volume loss in the posterior corpus callosum. The right image shows the LORETA image for the 10 Hz frequency domain in the eyes-opened condition as compared to the Life-span database. The regions of significant deficit compared to the normative sample are Brodmann Area (BA) 40 at inferior parietal lobe, BA 7 precuneus, superior parietal lobe, and BA 30/31 posterior cingulate. The total regions of decrease may reflect functionally related connections involved in numerous integrative processes, with an emphasis on language. The deficits shown in alpha extend to other frequencies with increased activity shown in the right hemisphere for nearly all frequency domains. (Cannon et al., 2011). Reprinted by permission of the publisher (Taylor & Francis Ltd, http://www.tand.co.uk/journals).

Figure 44 shows a saggital T1-weighted image of the brain. The volume of the posterior corpus callosum is significantly more disproportionate than would be expected. The LORETA image is for the theta frequency (5 Hz). The maximum deficit is shown at (x = -3, y = -39, z = 22) anterior cingulate gyrus with a z = -7.74. Deficits are also shown in the left insula. Theta power is increased in the bilateral prefrontal cortices, with higher increases shown in the right hemisphere.

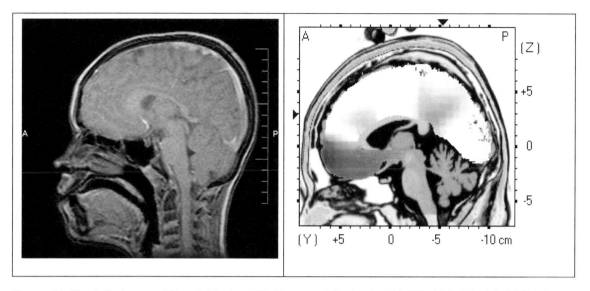

Figure 44: The left shows a T1-weighted sagittal image of the brain with TR: 63.7, TE: 1.6, DFOV: 24.0x 24.0 cm. Notice the volume in the posterior corpus callosum and posterior cingulate (also possibly affecting retrosplenial cortex). The right image is a sagittal view of LORETA current source density. Significant deficits in theta activity are shown in anterior (BA 24/32) and posterior cingulate (BA 31/7) cortices. Interestingly, increased alpha activity is shown in subgenual cingulate and medial/orbital prefrontal cortex. (Cannon et al., 2011). Reprinted by permission of the publisher (Taylor & Francis Ltd, http://www.tand.co.uk/journals).

Figure 45 shows a coronal T2-weighted image with emphasis on the temporal lobes. Atrophy is indicated in left temporal and bilateral frontal regions. The LORETA image for low-beta (15 Hz) is in a coronal view. The region of maximum decreased current source density is shown at left BA 40 in the inferior parietal lobe (x = -52, y = -32, z = 43) with z = -8.74.

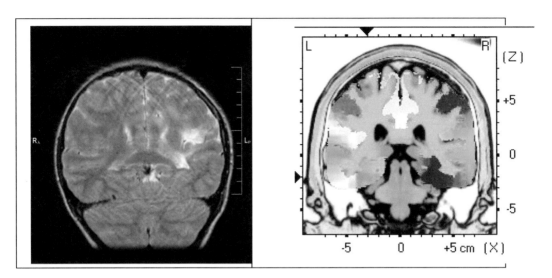

Figure 45: The left shows a coronal T2-weighted image of the brain highlighting Encephalomalacia in fronto-temporal regions (perisylvian regions), with Se: 11/11, TR: 3516.7, TE: 88.1, DFOV: 18.0 x 18.0 cm. The left hemisphere is shown on the right side of the image. The right image shows LORETA current source density deficits in mid beta activity in temporal areas, including BA 6, 7, 13, 20, 37, 30, 23 and hippocampus in the left hemisphere. (Cannon et al., 2011). Reprinted by permission of the publisher (Taylor & Francis Ltd, http://www.tand.co.uk/journals).

Figures 46 (ECB) and 47 (EOB) show 6 seconds of the raw EEG data collected from the patient. The EEG shows high amplitude theta activity at numerous locations over central and parietal locations. A notable asymmetry in the occipito-parietal areas is present, with faster activity shown in the right hemisphere. Increased alpha activity is shown in frontal leads, with deficient alpha shown posteriorly. Increased activity is shown in the right hemisphere for all frequency domains, with asymmetry seen across channels.

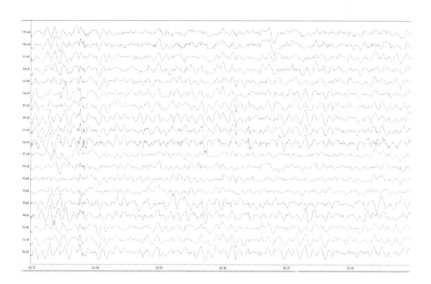

Figure 46: 6 seconds of raw EEG tracings in the eyes-closed resting. This record is scaled at 80mV. Excess beta is shown in posterior leads, especially concerning the right parietal region. The mean peak posterior dominant frequency is 8.80 µV with asymmetry present. High amplitude theta is shown throughout the record with higher levels appearing in the left hemisphere. (Cannon et al., 2011). Reprinted by permission of the publisher (Taylor & Francis Ltd, http://www.tand.co.uk/journals).

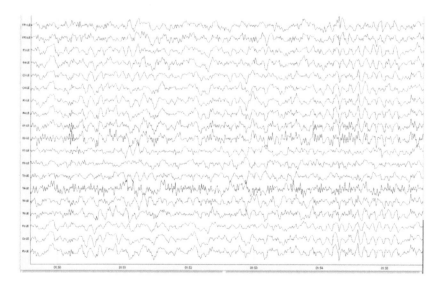

Figure 47: 6 seconds of raw EEG tracings for the eyes-opened recording. The record is scaled at 60mV. Increases in higher amplitude theta, which are more pronounced over the left hemisphere, are noted in addition to increased beta activity (faster activity over right temporal and occipital leads). Eye-movements are present in frontal leads in addition to slight EMG artifacts being present in the T4 tracing. (Cannon et al., 2011). Reprinted by permission of the publisher (Taylor & Francis Ltd, http://www.tand.co.uk/journals).

This was the first study of its kind to examine EEG current source density distributions in a pediatric case and compare them to the Lifespan database with MRI and neuropsychological validation. The neurocognitive sequelae associated with the MRI and EEG data include significant deficits in attention and self-regulation, working memory (and in fact all variants of memory), mathematics, visual-spatial organization and construction, orientation, as well as verbal acuity, production, and language processing in general. Importantly, both animal and human studies of developmental brain plasticity have indicated that the degree of sparing or recovery of functions following damage to the central nervous system depends upon the age at which an individual acquires the lesion.

Another important factor is lesion size, which shows a general relationship between lesion size and recovery, such that small neocortical lesions are associated with compensation mediated by brain regions ipsilateral to the side of injury, whereas larger lesions trigger compensatory changes in the contralateral hemisphere (Chugani, Muller, & Chugani, 1996). Functional reorganization or compensatory shifts with the increased EEG CSD activity may be evident in nearly all frequency domains in the right hemisphere. Similar increases in CSD are shown in the left hemisphere in non-affected regions.

Prefrontal and anterior cingulate regions that interact with parietal areas have been routinely demonstrated to represent core components of the circuitry executing top-down control of attentional processing (Gehring & Knight, 2002). The corpus callosum and posterior cingulate are important regions involved in functional integration processes (Bush et al., 1999; Bush et al., 2000; Whalen et al., 1998), including verbal/language functions as well as learning and memory in association with the hippocampus and medial temporal lobes (Zhou et al., 2008).

Encephalomalacic damage to numerous regions associated with language is present with the maximal deficits in all EEG frequency domains of the posterior parietal lobes, including left BA 40, posterior cingulate, and the precuneus (BA 31, 7, 23, 29, 30, 39, and 40). This identification may be directly associated with the deficits in the volume of the corpus callosum, with research showing that white matter activation of the isthmus is associated with gray matter activation in parietal lobes. This has important implications for multifunctional integration processes (Gawryluk, D'Arcy, Mazerolle, Brewer, & Beyea, 2010; Mazerolle et al., 2010).

Significant deficits in nearly all frequency domains are shown in left parieto-temporal regions, including auditory cortex and association areas (Heschl's gyrus transverse/superior temporal gyrus BA 41/42, BA 21/22) in the left hemisphere. EEG deficits identified in bilateral middle and medial prefrontal regions, including BA 6, 8, 9 10/47 and 11, indicating significant disruptions to bilateral prefrontal regions. BA 40, 39, and 2 show decrements in both hemispheres, with higher levels on the left side. The anterior cingulate gyrus shows deficits in both hemispheres, with higher levels in the right hemisphere (BA 24/32). Nearly all of the affected regions in this patient showed increased activity in control subjects during reading and word generation tasks (Liegeois et al., 2004). Importantly, concerning working memory and integrative functions associated with learning and encoding novel information, regions in the left dorsolateral prefrontal cortex involved in auditory and verbal working memory also showed significant deficits in activity (Grasby et al., 1993; Paulesu, Frith, & Frackowiak, 1993).

Changes in the EEG alpha rhythm may represent various important cognitive functions, including encoding, retrieval, and processing of information (Doppelmayr, Klimesch, Hodlmoser, et al., 2005; Doppelmayr, Klimesch, Sauseng, et al., 2005; Gruber et al., 2005; Sauseng, Klimesch, Doppelmayr, et al., 2005; Sauseng et al., 2006; Sauseng, Klimesch, Schabus, et al., 2005; Sauseng, Klimesch, Stadler, et al., 2005). Moreover, selective bands within the alpha frequency are also proposed to play a particular role in attention and working memory, with the lower alpha band (8 - 10 Hz) being associated with attention and the higher alpha band (10 - 12 Hz) being associated with working memory processes (Sauseng, Klimesch, Doppelmayr, et al., 2005). Alpha band power was also detected as having frontal (anterior cingulate) and limbic variants that are not susceptible to suppression by anxiolytics, unlike posterior alpha rhythms (Connemann, et al., 2005). Interestingly, the hallmark signature of EEG changes due to dementia of the Alzheimer's type involves a general slowing and decrease in alpha activity, which also shows an increase in theta activity. Cognitive decline is shown to be associated with changes in higher frequency domains in occipital and temporal regions, and such changes are shown to correlate with disease severity (Jeong, 2004). Posterial commissural fibers within the corpus callosum have shown the strongest correlation with the alpha frequency, such that the Isthmus and Tapetum in the superior occipital cortex show the highest positive association with the alpha frequency. Data suggests that the period of cortico-thalamocortical cycles may modulate the alpha frequency domain and that white matter architecture is associated more with the alpha frequency domain than with the neocortical region or grey matter (Valdes-Hernandez et al., 2010).

EEG LORETA, MRI, and neuropsychological data show excellent agreement in this particular case study. Therefore, comparing them with Lifespan database may be a valid tool for evaluating patient symptoms and correlating them with neural processes. Additionally, this type of analysis is important to differential diagnosis aimed at measuring treatment efficacy and developing multidisciplinary treatment models. When compared to the Lifespan database, the LORETA analyses for this patient identify multifocal deficits in regions also identified by MRI. We know that although the specific functions of the EEG and reasons for specific deficits in specific frequencies due to damage remain uncertain, they are involved in cognitive and attentive processes as well as disruptions in specific regions and associated EEG frequency domains associated with psychiatric syndromes (Coutin-Churchman et al., 2003; Hughes, 1995, 1996). Interestingly, social and daily functioning activities are minimally impaired in this patient. He interacts appropriately with siblings and peers, although difficulty with remembering names presents significant challenges. Comparison to a control group is often a challenge in the clinical setting.

Therefore, the Lifespan database offers a potential method to facilitate clinical data that are more comprehensive in order to serve the patient better. One important limitation of the current data is that we cannot discern whether the Encephalomalacia is an end-point or progressive in nature. The cumulative data show agreement between MRI, EEG LORETA, and neuropsychological data. Further multidisciplinary studies of this type are needed to improve our understanding of neurocognitive mechanisms in pediatric populations. The current findings also stress the importance of correlating patient symptoms with neurophysiological and neuroanatomical data, which is the primary goal of neuropsychology.

3.8: Summary

LORETA and qEEG provide a means to study fundamental mechanisms of neural activity in normal as well as psychiatric populations. These methods can be used to determine treatment efficacy and monitor changes in the brain that occur because of neurofeedback, pharmacological, and psychotherapeutic interventions. In this brief summary of depression, anxiety, substance use disorders, and Attention Deficit-Hyperactivity Disorder, it is clear that each disorder is in some aspects notably unique and in other aspects similar in both frequency and regional deficits. Functional connectivity and network analyses are important directions for studying these syndromes and dynamic processes involved in associated neurocognitive sequelae. qEEG and LORETA in combination with other methods (e.g., fMRI and PET) can be used to expand on the structural data. This may provide a means to advance our understanding of frequency specific functions and insights into the comorbidity rates, which can be very high for these four disorders. Our knowledge of the specific functions and origins of the EEG still involves much uncertainty; thus, EEG and LORETA, in combination with other neuroimaging techniques, can serve an important role in improving this knowledge base.

CHAPTER 4

LORETA Neurofeedback

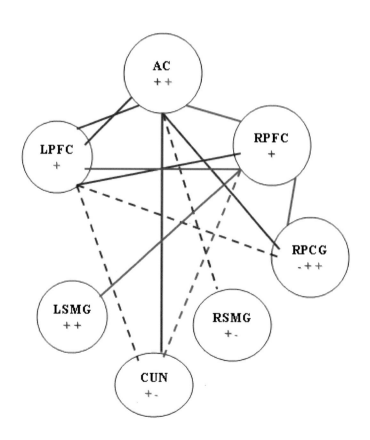

CHAPTER 4

LORETA Neurofeedback

LORETA neurofeedback (LNFB) was developed by Dr. Marco Congedo at the Brain Research and Neuropsychology laboratory at the University of Tennessee, Knoxville (Congedo et al., 2004). It was my pleasure to work with both Dr. Congedo and Dr. Joel Lubar in this early implementation and subsequent work. In the most basic sense, LORETA neurofeedback monitors the current source density, calculated by the LORETA algorithm in real time for a specific cluster of voxels or region of training (ROT) in the intracranial space. This activity is set to covary with auditory and visual displays to provide feedback to the patient/participant. Specific cognitive/attentional/self-regulatory processes are engaged to change the level of current source density in the specified region of training (ROT). In conventional neurofeedback, electroencephalographic (EEG) activity is recorded at a particular scalp location. The physiological measurements are extrapolated from the signal and converted into auditory stimuli or visual objects that animatedly co-vary with the magnitude of a specified brain frequency or frequency band. Likewise, LNFB sets the physiological signal to correlate with a continuous feedback signal; however, the physiological signal is defined as the current density in the specified ROT. This allows the continuous feedback signal to become a function of the intracranial current density and to covary with it. Figure 48 shows the regions of training and populations (or case studies) our laboratory has employed to date.

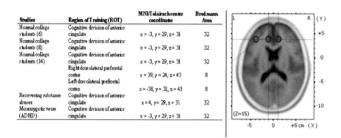

Studies	Region of Training (ROT)	MNI/Talairach center coordinates	Brodmann Area
Normal college students (6)	Cognitive division of anterior cingulate	x = -3, y = 29, z = 31	32
Normal college students (8)	Cognitive division of anterior cingulate	x = -3, y = 29, z = 31	32
Normal college students (14)	Cognitive division of anterior cingulate	x = -3, y = 29, z = 31	32
	Right dorsolateral prefrontal cortex	x = 39, y = 24, z = 43	8
	Left dorsolateral prefrontal cortex	x = -38, y = 31, z = 43	8
Recovering substance abuser	Cognitive division of anterior cingulate	x = 4, y = 29, z = 31	32
Monozygotic twins (ADHD)	Cognitive division of anterior cingulate	x = -3, y = 29, z = 31	32

Figure 48: Studies of LNFB

Participants are prepared for EEG recording using a measure of the head circumference and the distance between the nasion and inion to determine the appropriate cap size for recording (e.g., 58*1.0 = 5.8, 36*1.0 = 3.6) and placement of the two frontal electrodes (FP1 & FP2). The head is measured and marked prior to baseline recording and each subsequent recording across sessions to maintain consistency. The ears and forehead are cleaned for recording with a mild abrasive gel (NuPrep) to remove any oil and dirt from the skin. After fitting the caps, each electrode site is injected with electrogel and prepared so that impedances between individual electrodes and each ear are < 10 KΩ. An important consideration for impedances is that if not all electrodes reach the desired level, the difference between electrodes should be minimized. In our studies thus far, LNFB training has been conducted using the 19-leads standard international 10/20 system. The data are collected and stored with a band pass set at 0.5 - 64.0 Hz at a rate of 256 samples per second using the Deymed Truscan Acquisition system (Deymed Diagnostics).

All recordings and sessions are conducted in a comfortably lit, sound attenuated room at the University of Tennessee, Knoxville. In all studies, lighting and temperature are held constant for the duration of the experiment. We also maintain the same research assistant per participant throughout the training sessions. Importantly, after sufficient training, even the most novice research assistant or technician can complete each session in approximately fifty minutes. The total capping time is less than 15 minutes for most newly trained research assistants.

The range of sessions in each of the studies conducted by our lab is between twenty and thirty-three. Each session in these early studies composed of pre and post eyes-closed and eyes-opened baselines and four four-minute training rounds conducted three times per week (Cannon, 2007; Cannon et al., 2009; Cannon et al., 2007; Cannon & Lubar, 2008; Cannon, Lubar, Gerke, Thornton, Hutchens, & McCammon, 2006; Cannon, Sokhadze, Lubar, & Baldwin, 2008). Participant reports have directly influenced the length of training rounds and sessions. Most participants reported boredom and irritation (discomfort) after five minutes. In the studies conducted thus far, we trained individuals to increase 14 -18 Hz (low-beta) power activity in specific clusters of voxels. The center voxel for each cluster is shown in Figure 48.

The AC cluster contains 7 voxels, the right prefrontal cluster contains 4, and the left prefrontal cluster contains 3. Currently, we are conducting clinical trials for LNFB in the right and left precuneus. An important behavioral function utilized in early sessions with all individuals is shaping. Since an operant response must occur at some minimum frequency to be reinforced, we perform a preliminary session of shaping with each participant in order to ascertain the ability of the participant to meet the criteria set forth and obtain a minimum reinforcement effect (points $\geq$ 10 per minute) in the standardized protocol. During this session, the participants are made aware of artifact production and instructed to control tongue and eye movements, eye-blinks, and muscle activity of the forehead, neck, and jaws. This enables the subjects to become aware of mental activity required to minimize the production of extra-cranial artifacts (EMG, EOG, etc.) during the sessions.

Participants are then set for the reward protocol at the ROT; however, it is important for the participant or patient to score a minimum of 10 points in one session, otherwise reinforcement will be more difficult and will influence the likelihood of successful completion of the protocol and the operant conditioning procedure. Thresholds are then set and maintained for each participant throughout the training protocol. Participants are required to suppress Electrooculogram (EOG) activity to < 15.0 (Microvolts) and Electromyogram (EMG) activity to < 6.0 (Microvolts) while simultaneously increasing current source density at the Region of Training (ROT).

Our research studies have been conducted using Deymed Truscan hardware and software and as such, the following examples of the protocol setup illustrate these particular software settings. Figure 49 shows the LNFB protocol setup in the older version of the software.

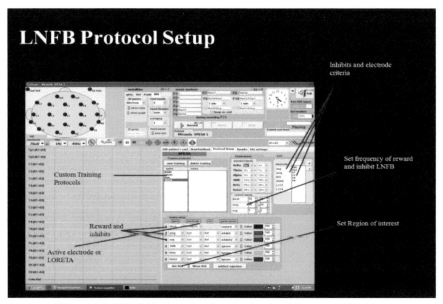

Figure 49: LNFB Protocol setup in Deymed Truscan System.

In newer versions, many of the options are automatically entered by button-clicks. In the image from left to right are the training protocols that can be fixed for a group or an individual patient, the reward and inhibit selections, active electrode or LORETA ROT, and to the right the linear combinations of channels to fit the inhibit criteria. Figure 50 (next page) shows the LORETA ROT setup. The displayed screen becomes available once the user defines that LORETA will be used as the reward stimuli (ROT). The user can then enter the x, y, and z coordinates for the center voxel of the ROT. Figure 51 (next page) depicts the LORETA image showing the location of the region of training by clicking the view ROI in the Deymed interface.

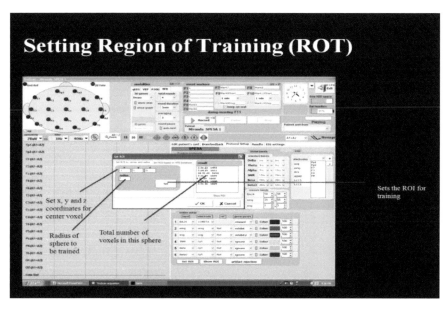

Figure 50: Setting region of training (ROT)

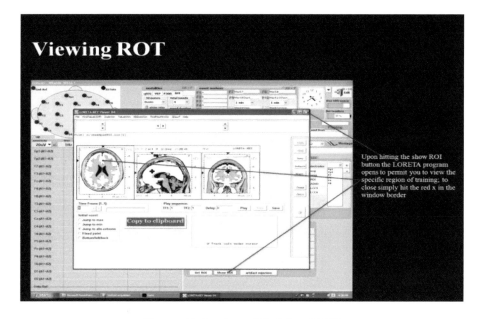

Figure 51: Region of Training (ROT)

The participants in our studies are provided visual and auditory feedback. Points are achieved when 1 - 3 Hz activity decreases simultaneously in a linear combination of six frontal channels, FP1, FP2, F3, F4, F7, F8 and when 35 - 55 Hz activity decreases in a linear combination of six temporal and occipital channels, T3, T4, T5, T6, O1, and O2, while increasing current source density (14 - 18 Hz) in the specific ROT. Maintaining the condition for 0.75 seconds achieves one point. The auditory stimuli provide both positive and negative reinforcement, an unpleasant splat sound when the conditions are not met, and a pleasant tone when they are met. Similarly, the visual stimuli are activated when the criteria are being met, e.g., a car or a spaceship driving faster and straighter. Alternatively, a slower car driving in the wrong lane or the spaceship flying slow and crooked occur when the criteria are not being met. The participants can also see the score needed to meet the criteria in a small window of the game screen. Subsequent chapters will discuss the specific features of reinforcement and reward concerning neurofeedback (operant conditioning) methods in more detail in order to bring clarity to this process.

4.1: Clinical Applications

LORETA Neurofeedback offers an exciting potential for the treatment of psychological syndromes, trauma related injuries, as well as performance enhancing drug use among athletes, performers, and various stress or anxiety provoking professions. One of the more important theoretical implications is the potential to influence cortical regions associated to produce changes in self-concept, self-image, and self-perception in order to change behavior. This is an area of concentrated study in our laboratory. In the following sections, I will provide examples of LORETA neurofeedback and the neurophysiological changes that occur because of this training. Numerous features of LORETA/sLORETA are worth exploring, including coherence, phase synchrony, frequency specific changes, cross-frequency correlations, and network analyses by temporal correlations and partial correlation procedures. Some of the data presented in this section are still in the process of theoretical consideration; however, I believe the data applies to the neuroscience of EEG and the brain inclusively.

4.2: Statistical Considerations

A wide range of statistical procedures is used to report neurofeedback results. Typically, pre and post baselines may be compared using paired t-tests. Learning curves may be plotted and evaluated using linear models or time series techniques. One of the more important considerations in reporting neurofeedback results are the correlations (e.g., interdependence) between rounds, sessions and even baselines. This is also an important consideration for any type of repeated measurement using EEG or LORETA or other neuroimaging method. ANOVA procedures maintain the assumption of independent observations (x and y are not related). Neurofeedback violates this assumption such that each session is dependent on and correlated with the prior session as are each round within each session. In basic terms, an analysis-of-variance (ANOVA) model can be written as a linear model. The resulting equation predicts the response as a linear function of both parameters and design variables. Once models are expressed in the framework of linear models, hypothesis tests are expressed in expressions of a linear function of the parameters. Each fixed effect is a single variable or combination of variables. Fitting mixed linear models to data enables us to make statistical inferences about the data and control for these typical violations (Wackerly, 2002).

A mixed linear model is a generalization of the standard linear model used in the GLM procedure, the generalization being that the data are permitted to exhibit correlation and nonconstant variability. The mixed linear model, therefore, provides the flexibility of modeling the means of the data (as in the standard linear model) as well as the variances and covariances. This is very important to functional network analytic procedures and determining the influence of the region of training on specific regional neuronal locations (i.e., the strengthening or changing of network connectivity). The primary assumptions underlying the analyses performed by mixed procedures are as follows: The data are normally distributed (Gaussian). The means (expected values) of the data are linear in terms of a certain set of parameters. The variances and covariances of the data are in terms of a different set of parameters, and they exhibit a structure matching one of available models.

Since Gaussian data can be modeled entirely in terms of their means and variances/covariances, the two sets of parameters in a mixed linear model actually specify the complete probability distribution of the data. The parameters of the mean model are referred to as fixed-effects parameters, and the parameters of the variance-covariance model are referred to as covariance parameters. The fixed-effects parameters are associated with known explanatory variables, as in the standard linear model. These variables can be either qualitative (as in the traditional analysis of variance) or quantitative (as in standard linear regression). However, the covariance parameters distinguish the mixed linear model from the standard linear model (Kackar, 1984; Neter, 2006; Wackerly, 2002). The need for covariance parameters arises quite frequently in applications, the following being the two most typical scenarios: The experimental units on which the data are measured can be grouped into clusters, and the data from a common cluster are correlated. Repeated measurements are taken on the same experimental unit, and these repeated measurements are correlated or exhibit variability that changes (Neter, 2006).

The mixed model provides various covariance structures to handle the previous two scenarios. The most common of these structures arises from the use of random-effects parameters, which are additional unknown random variables (typically in neuroscience subjects/patients) assumed to influence the variability of the data. The variances of the random-effects parameters, commonly known as variance components become the covariance parameters for this particular structure. Thus, the mixed procedure fits not only these traditional variance component models but numerous other covariance structures as well. Mixed models fit the preselected structure to the data using the method of restricted maximum likelihood (REML) also known as residual maximum likelihood. The mixed procedure computes several different statistics suitable for generating hypothesis tests and confidence intervals. Compound symmetry assumes the same variance for each measurement and the same covariance between any two measurements. In consideration of these assumptions, it is practical that the correlations between measurements taken closer together in time would be higher compared to measurements taken further apart in time (Kackar, 1984; Lahiri, 1995; Prasad, 1990; Wackerly, 2002).

The residual variance is a part of the mixed model and can feasibly be profiled out of the likelihood estimates. This means solving systematically for the most advantageous expression and putting it back into the likelihood formula (Wolfinger, Tobias, & Sall, 1994). This reduces the number of optimization parameters by one and improves convergence properties. The mixed procedure profiles the residual variance out of the log likelihood whenever it appears reasonable to do so. In many situations, the best approach is to use *likelihood-based* methods, exploiting the assumption that G and R (covariance structure matrices) are normally distributed (Hartley & Rao, 1967; Harville, 1977; Jennrich & Schluchter, 1986; Laird & Ware, 1982; Patterson & Thompson, 1971). Thus, reporting the effects of Neurotherapy requires a sophisticated adjustment to typical statistical procedures. This reflects both the complexity of the brain and the treatment modality used to influence or change its functional parameters. Figure 52 shows a graphical representation of the relationship between network assemblages. Training in the AC produces dramatic and statistically significant increases in the bilateral prefrontal cortices.

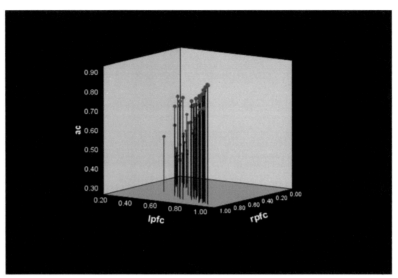

Figure 52: The degree to which the increase in a specific frequency (14 - 18 Hz) in the AC or (ROT) influences increase or decrease in (14 - 18 Hz) the other regions of interest within the covariance structure, controlling for the effects of all other ROIs in the particular study. (The strengthening of a network). The fixed effects the AC or (ROT) produces in the other ROIs within the covariance structure. (The learning effect within the network).

4.3: Examples

Neurofeedback operates under the auspices of neural plasticity. As indicated in earlier sections and a large literature base in both human and animal studies, environmental conditions do produce effects on neuronal structure and synchronous functionality. In this section, I will cover basic findings of studies examining the anterior cingulate and dorsolateral prefrontal cortices. Pilot data guided the selection of the region for training and the specific frequency on which we should concentrate. When training the anterior cingulate gyrus, these two notions required intensive exploration. We elected to train low-beta power based on the results from conventional neurofeedback studies. In pilot data, we also trained the theta frequency (4 - 7Hz) in the AC. Participants were able to increase this frequency; however, as the time-in-reward increased, so did excessive tear production. This was not associated with an emotional change, as reported by the participants. It did influence the ability to continue training during the session. We elected to discontinue the theta and increase low-beta. All participants were able to adapt and continue with the training successfully. Thus, both frequency and region play a

therefore, caution and careful attention to these factors is vital to the L

short, we do not have sufficient knowledge about frequency specific fu

or other intracranial training (rt-fMRI) may influence.

Following the pilot study, we utilized LNFB with eight undergraduate students. Specifically, we trained them to increase 14 - 18 Hz (low-beta) power in the anterior cingulate gyrus ($x = -31$, $y = 29$, $Z = 31$). The most impressive result was the substantial increase in working memory and processing speed scores (~11 points), as shown in Figure 53.

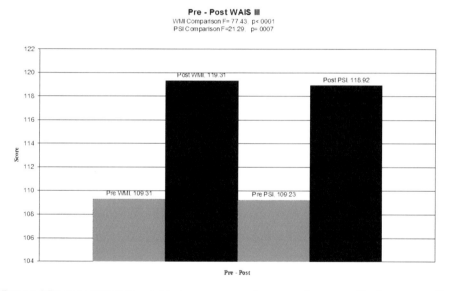

Pre - Post WAIS III
WMI Comparison F= 77.43; p< 0001
PSI Comparison F=21.29; p= 0007

Figure 53: Pre and Post contrast in working memory and processing speed index scores for the WAIS-III. For the 3 groups (AC, left and right prefrontal), there is a significant effect of LNFB training. (Cannon, Congedo, Lubar & Hutchens, 2009). International Journal of Neuroscience by TAYLOR & FRANCIS INC. Reproduced with permission of TAYLOR & FRANCIS INC. in the format Journal via Copyright Clearance Center.

This result was similar (~10 points) in later studies on LNFB in the right and left dorsolateral prefrontal cortices. Of particular interest is the apparent involvement of the AC in all cognitive processes associated with working memory and processing speed, as shown in Figure 54 (next page) , whereas the left and right prefrontal appear to have

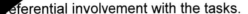

eferential involvement with the tasks.

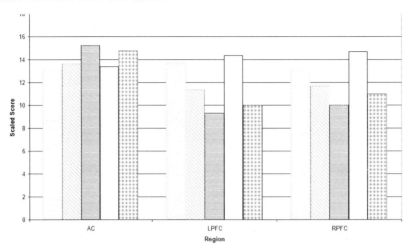

Figure 54: Post training scaled scores for each ROT group. Interestingly, the AC shows an apparent involvement in all measures while the left and right show apparent preference toward coding and symbol search. This is an observation of the training and not a statistically proven effect. (Cannon, Congedo, Lubar & Hutchens, 2009). International Journal of Neuroscience by TAYLOR & FRANCIS INC. Reproduced with permission of TAYLOR & FRANCIS INC. in the format Journal via Copyright Clearance Center.

We did obtain subjective reports from all subjects in AC and right and left prefrontal training. Notably, the AC group reported more mental direction toward attention and working memory processes, while the left group reported a higher frequency of time toward attention, specifically with utilizing working memory somewhat less, and the right group utilized a working memory, visual processes, and mental verbalization (i.e., mental verbalization with the game or self). In the course of our experiments, we have used LNFB with recovering substance abusers, ADHD, and non-clinical participants and reported both topographical as well as connectivity changes within the intracranial space (Cannon et al., 2009; Cannon & Lubar, 2008; Cannon et al., 2007; Cannon et al., 2006; Cannon et al., 2008). Figure 55 (next page) shows the learning curve for the AC and its effects on the right and left PFC.

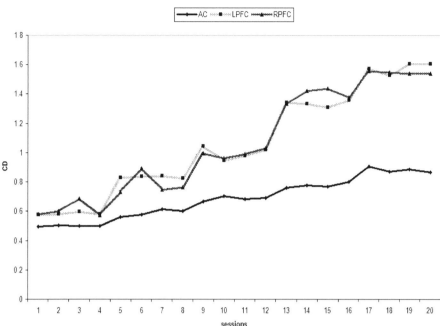

Learning Curves for AC as a result of training in AC, LPFC, RPFC

Figure 55: Learning curve in the AC group and its effects on the LPFC and RPFC. The learning curve in the AC is significant and its relationship with both left and right prefrontal cortices is significant. As the activity in the AC increases, so do these bilateral prefrontal regions. (Cannon, Congedo, Lubar & Hutchens, 2009). International Journal of Neuroscience by TAYLOR & FRANCIS INC. Reproduced with permission of TAYLOR & FRANCIS INC. in the format Journal via Copyright Clearance Center.

Importantly, participants were able to sustain and increase CSD in the AC with notable changes in working memory and processing speed. Figure 56 (page 131) is undoubtedly one of the most difficult images to interpret from the LNFB experiments. In the figure from top to bottom and left to right are the partial correlations and GLM results for seven regions of interest, as influenced by the training in each of three ROT. The image shows the trained frequency, alpha-1, alpha-2, delta, theta, and beta, respectively. The solid lines indicate positive relationships while the dashed lines indicate negative relationships. Only correlations or GLM effects significant at .01 are plotted in the image. It is reasonable to consider this a layering effect within the cortical matter, with the assumption that brain stem and thalamic regions underlie this activity. Therefore, we are not certain whether thalamo-cortical circuits are at work here and, given the brain stem reticular formation is responsible for higher frequency activity in the cortex as well as possibly all frequency activity, further work needs to be done to understand these mechanisms fully.

Additionally, the results of the studies involving the AC produce very similar results as real-time fMRI training (Weiskopf, Mathiak, et al., 2004; Weiskopf, Scharnowski, et al., 2004). In conclusion, LNFB has the potential to influence regions within the neocortex as well as limbic areas that are thought to be involved in numerous psychopathologies, as noted earlier.

Figure 56 (next page): The figure contains the correlation and GLM results for each frequency, left to right and top to bottom: (a) TF; (b) alpha 1; (c) alpha 2; (d) delta; (e) Theta; (f) beta. The partial correlation results are shown with lines; each figure represents the relationship of each ROT with each of the ROIs while controlling for the effects of the other five ROIs. Thus, the lines indicate a 1:1 correlation, controlling for the effects of the remaining ROIs. The red lines represent training in the AC; the blue lines represent training in the LPFC; and the green lines represent training in the RPFC. The solid lines indicate positive relationships that meet statistical criteria. The dashed lines indicate negative relationships that meet the statistical criteria. The GLM results are reported in the same color scheme: AC = red symbols; LPFC = blue symbols; RPFC = green symbols; + = increased activity effects for the ROI in relation to ROT; - = decreased activity effects for the ROI in relation to ROT. The GLM procedure shows the increase or decrease of each ROI in relation to the specific ROT (i.e., the learning effect within the network), while the partial correlation procedure shows the strengthening of the network. (Cannon, Congedo, Lubar & Hutchens, 2009). International Journal of Neuroscience by TAYLOR & FRANCIS INC. Reproduced with permission of TAYLOR & FRANCIS INC. in the format Journal via Copyright Clearance Center.

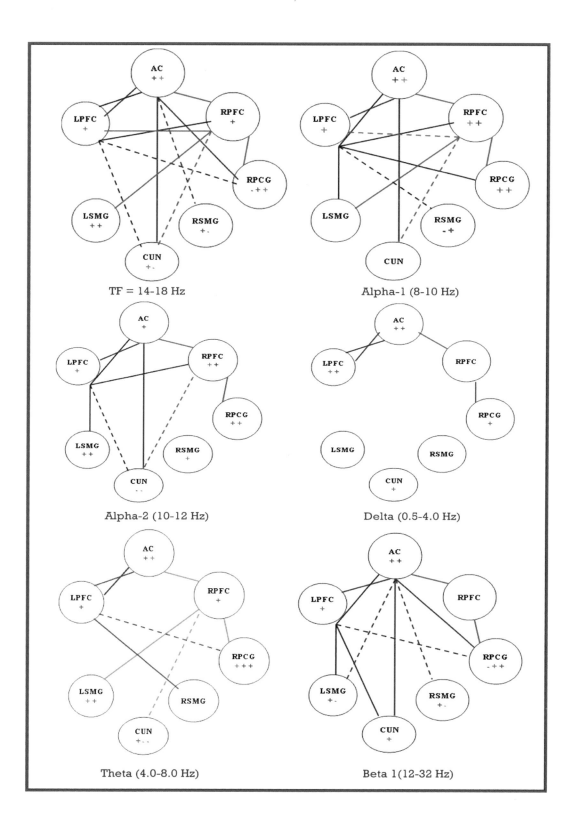

4.4: Summary

LORETA neurofeedback, like traditional neurofeedback methods, utilizes principles of operant conditioning. The LORETA algorithm is calculated in real-time and is set to covary with auditory or visual stimuli that provide feedback to the individual. Thus far, several studies have demonstrated the human beings can learn to change the activity in specific regions of the cortex and this operant behavior does influence network connectivity within the brain. LNFB and rt-fMRI feedback arrive to similar results. Importantly, LNFB offers the potential to influence regions of the brain that might not otherwise be accessible by conventional neurofeedback techniques. This is important to numerous psychopathologies, given that limbic and medial cortical regions are thought to play an important role in specific symptoms (e.g., orbital frontal, limbic, and posterior cingulate cortices). LNFB studies have shown significant improvements in working memory and processing speed scores and as such may suggest an important method to improve performance of normal individuals as well. There is certainly much work to be done. One of our current studies is a randomized controlled double-blind intervention study of LNFB in the anterior cingulate and left precuneus conducted with ADHD adults. We are also performing clinical intervention trials of LNFB in the precuneus in SUD with adjunct cognitive, affective, and perceptual mechanisms. Combination of these methods may substantially improve our understanding of self-regulation and the components necessary to develop and maintain this poorly defined construct.

CHAPTER 5

A Brief Review of Brodmann Areas and Functional Neuroanatomy

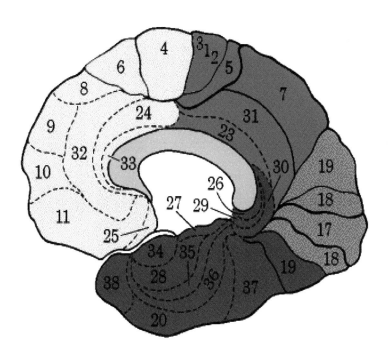

CHAPTER 5

A Brief Review of Brodmann Areas and Functional Neuroanatomy

This section assumes that users will be conducting studies with LORETA or will utilize it in a NF treatment paradigm. The review is not inclusive by any means; however, it is my hope that the reader can formulate hypotheses based on empirical neuroscientific data and obtain a general knowledge of regional function, neuroanatomy, and neurocognitive mechanisms of interest in known psychopathologies as well as normative functioning. This section will provide a brief review of Brodmann areas (BA) and functional neuroanatomy in addition to network connectivity. This review will provide the reader a basic knowledge of region and known activation patterns found in neuroimaging studies, including EEG LORETA.

The reader is also provided numerous references to functional connectivity studies that examine the default network and resting state networks in the human brain. This area of research is extremely important as it increases our knowledge of distributed networks in the brain during both rest and specific cognitive tasks. Recently, a concentrated area of study has demonstrated that it is feasible to examine the EEG CSD activity in the default network and resting state networks, respectively. Importantly, this section considers our current knowledge of the human brain and its limitations. We are still in the early perinatal period; therefore, conclusions made today will undoubtedly be refuted tomorrow and as

135

such, I encourage all scientists to operate with this limitation in mind. Thus, as experts we are bound to the integrity of our science and our conclusions.

Table 1 provides the international standards for anatomical brain research.

FOREBRAIN	*Diencephalon*	Epithalamus, thalamus, hypothalamus, subthalamus
	Telencephalon	Cerebral cortex, olfactory bulb, amygdala, septal region, fornix, basal ganglia [globus palidus, striatum (caudate and putamen)]
MIDBRAIN	*Mesencephalon*	Tectum, pretectal region, superior colliculus, inferior colliculus
		Cerebral peduncle
HINDBRAIN	*Myelencephalon*	Medulla oblongata, vestibular nuclei, cochlear nuclei, medullary reticular formation, raphe nuclei, solitary nucleus, ovary complex
	Metencephalon	Pons, cerebellum

Table 1: International standards for anatomical brain research.

There are three principle divisions of the brain, the forebrain, midbrain, and hindbrain. The telencephalon is the most rostral (anterior or toward the oral/nasal region) portion of the brain and is primarily composed of the cerebral hemispheres (cerebrum) and their ancillaries. The cerebral cortices consist of an outer cortex of gray matter and an inner bulk of white matter. The gray matter is a dense collection of cell bodies, whereas the white matter is formed by myelinated and unmyelinated axons linking neuronal populations (Hanaway, 1998).

The Diencephalon is the second, interior part of the forebrain. All information entering or leaving the telencephalon must past through this region, which is situated in the brain stem, specifically at the head of the brain stem linking the cerebral cortex with lower (notice I did not use the term more primitive) brain-stem structures. The diencephalon is not formed by a system of fiber pathways; instead, it is composed primarily of gray matter and is implicated in various central nervous system functions. The components within the diencephalon are composed of individual specialized nuclei and dense concentrations of gray matter that perform differential functional roles. The mesencephalon is between the forebrain and hindbrain and is the smallest portion of the brain stem. At its central core is the mesencephalic tegmentum. The tegmentum surrounds the cerebral aqueduct, which is a thin canal linking the third and fourth ventricles. Neurons in the midbrain reticular formation have long branching axons that bifurcate and run ascending or descending to telencephalon or medulla locations. This region is known to play a vital role in attention, alerting, and orienting (Rosenberg, 1998). The superior colliculus or optic tectum in the midbrain and its downstream brain-stem-gaze center circuits form robust pattern generator to coordinate movements of various body parts to orient the gaze in all the vertebrate species (Isa & Sasaki, 2002; Isaacman, Poirier, Loiselle, & Schutzman, 2002; Sparks, 2002). Thus, the basic system that controls orienting behavior operates at the brainstem level and under the control of higher order structures, such as fronto-parietal cortices and basal ganglia. Two major visual pathways are known to exist. The first projects direct connections to the superior colliculus (retino-tectal or extrageniculate visual pathway), and the second reaches the cerebral cortex via the lateral geniculate nucleus (geniculo-striatal visual pathway).

One important region often neglected in the discussion of reward and reinforcement is the ventral tegmental area (VTA). It is implicated in numerous appetitive, sexual, and rewarding behaviors. Importantly, the VTA's primary focus is on reward and pleasurable activities since the dopaminergic cell bodies are found here and the VTA projects to mesolimbic area (e.g., septal and medial frontal and limbic regions) (Broderick, 1992; Lodge & Grace, 2006; Shankaranarayana Rao, Raju, & Meti, 1998). To illustrate the VTA's importance in pleasurable activity, in the following sections, I will discuss research that evaluated orgasm in male and female participants.

FMRI research on brain regions activated during orgasm in females with spinal cord injuries included the hypothalamic paraventricular nucleus, amygdala, accumbens-bed nucleus of the stria terminalis-preoptic area, hippocampus, basal ganglia (especially putamen), cerebellum, and anterior cingulate, insular, parietal and frontal cortices, and lower brainstem (central gray, mesencephalic reticular formation, and the nucleus of the solitary tract in the medulla oblongata (Alexander & Rosen, 2008). The authors concluded that the vagus nerve provides a spinal cord-bypass pathway for vaginal cervical sensibility and that activation of this pathway can produce analgesia and orgasm. Another study of sexual stimulation of the clitoris (compared to rest) showed significant increase in regional cerebral blood flow (rCBF) in the left secondary and right dorsal primary somatosensory cortex. This demonstrated the first account of neocortical processing of sexual clitoral information. On the contrary, when compared with the controls, orgasm was associated with profound rCBF decreases in the neocortex, namely the left lateral orbitofrontal cortex, inferior temporal gyrus, and anterior temporal pole (Opsomer & Guerit, 1991). It has been posited that decreased blood flow in the left lateral orbitofrontal cortex was indicative of behavioral disinhibition during orgasm in women and that decreased activity in the temporal lobe was related to high sexual arousal. Additionally, cerebellar nuclei seemed to be involved in orgasm-specific muscle contractions while activation of the ventral midbrain and right caudate nucleus seemed to indicate a role of dopaminergic pathways in female sexual arousal and orgasm (Komisaruk & Whipple, 2005).

Brain regions involved in male ejaculation show primary activation in the mesodiencephalic transition zone, including the VTA, which is shown active in rewarding behaviors. Other regions of increased activity included the central tegmental field, zona incerta, subparafascicular nucleus, and the ventroposterior, midline, and intralaminar thalamic nuclei. Activity in the lateral putamen and adjoining parts of the claustrum was also increased. Salient activity increase in the cortex was restricted to Brodmann areas 7/40, 18, 21, 23, and 47 in the right hemisphere. These findings are different from rodent studies in that the amygdala and adjacent entorhinal cortex did not show increased activation. Thus, the authors concluded that the cerebellum, in conjunction with the other above-mentioned regions, plays an important role in ejaculatory processes. The VTA plays an important role in sexual behavior, maternal behavior, reward, and addictive disorders. It is also important for the processing of self and social mechanisms (Kenny, Chartoff, Roberto, Carlezon, & Markou, 2009; Laviolette & van der Kooy, 2004; Nikulina, Miczek, & Hammer, 2005; Schumann, Michaeli, & Yaka, 2009). The VTA is mentioned in this context due to its important role in reward and pleasurable activities.

Considerable emphasis has been placed on the putative role of nucleus accumbens and dopamine systems in appetitive motivation and positive reinforcement. It has been suggested that dopamine (DA) systems mediate the "hedonic" effects of stimuli that act as positive reinforcers, such as food, water, sex, and drugs of abuse. Some appetitive motivated conditions, including lever pressing for food or administration of drugs of abuse, can increase nucleus accumbens DA release. This DA release has been suggested to mediate the pleasurable effect of reinforcing stimuli. In turn, an implicit assumption of this line of reasoning is that the "hedonia" induced by nucleus accumbens DA release directly mediates the process of positive reinforcement. Finally, it has been suggested that DA antagonists produce a state of "anhedonia", which has been interpreted to mean that DA antagonists blunt the positive reinforcing properties of hedonic stimuli literally by blocking the "goodness" of stimuli such as food. DA antagonists interfere with aversively motivated behavior, such as active avoidance. Moreover, various aversive or stressful conditions have been shown to increase accumbens DA release or metabolism. It is possible to state empirically that DA systems are involved in behavioral processes related to both positive and negative reinforcement, yet such a conclusion does not provide support for a hedonia-based hypothesis of dopaminergic involvement in reinforcement (Fibiger & Phillips, 1988; Fricchione & Stefano, 2005; Ikemoto, 2007; Jerlhag et al., 2006; Lawrence, Evans, & Lees, 2003).

The existing studies, other than amphetamine studies, provide no evidence that the involvement of DA systems in emotion is selective for "hedonia", "euphoria", or other such emotions with positive valence (Drevets et al., 2001). Evidence indicates that impairments in dopaminergic function may disrupt some aspects of motivation, yet leave others intact. Active avoidance and escape are both aspects of aversive motivation, yet DA antagonists can impair avoidance at doses that do not impair escape. Impairments in positively reinforced lever pressing can be produced at doses of DA antagonists that do not impair relatively simple approach responses. Doses of DA antagonists that impair positively reinforced instrumental behavior can have little effect on the consumatory response to the stimulus that is used as the reinforcer.

Considerable evidence indicates that DA in striatum and nucleus accumbens is involved in aspects of motor function. Thus, it is possible that interference with DA systems impairs instrumental behavior because of disruptions of motor function. Thus, there are still many unanswered questions concerning the role of dopamine in motivation and emotion, in addition to the effects of self-reinforcement as applied to human beings (Di Chiara, 1995; Hull, Du, Lorrain, & Matuszewich, 1995; Mitchell & Gratton, 1994; Salamone, 1994; Satoh, Nakai, Sato, & Kimura, 2003; Volkow et al., 2002; Wang, Volkow, & Fowler, 2002; Wise, 2004).

Korbinian Brodmann published the most generally accepted and enduring cytoarchitectural map of the human cerebral cortex in 1908. The respective nomenclature ranges from 1 to 52 labeled as Brodmann Areas (BA). Several of the original BA have been subdivided further and named by divisions. The anterior cingulate gyrus is a very good example of such a subdivision (Devinsky, Morrell, & Vogt, 1995). One of the more complex issues in neuroimaging studies is that there is a very high degree of overlap in regional activation patterns during different cognitive, emotional, and attentional tasks. Thus, the human brain is perhaps best described as a complex system of complex systems. In essence, a reductionist or strict localization approach to neural functions may hinder the discovery of complex functional systems, based in synchrony, coherency, and functional connectivity. Indeed the mechanisms and specificity of their functions are the greatest of enigmas.

In a geometric sense, the cerebral cortex is vast sheet of neurons through which any number of interconnections and interactions are possible (Griffin, 1994). The cortex is traditionally divided into four general regions or lobes. The frontal lobe is the most anterior and is separated from the rest of the cortex by the central fissure (also called the Rolandic fissure). Directly posterior to the frontal lobe is the parietal lobe and the lateral fissure (also called the Sylvian fissure) inferiorly bounds the parietal lobe. The parietal lobe is between the frontal and occipital lobes and is situated above the temporal lobe. On its lateral aspect, its most rostral gyrus, the postcentral gyrus, is the primary somesthetic area to which primary somatosensory information is directed from the contralateral half of the body (Hanaway, 1998).

The remainder of the parietal lobe, separated from the postcentral gyrus by the postcentral sulcus, is subdivided by the intraparietal sulcus into the superior and inferior parietal lobules. The superior parietal lobe is an association area involved in somatosensory function, whereas the latter is separated into the supramarginal gyrus, which integrates auditory, visual, and somatosensory information, and the angular gyrus, which receives visual input. On its medial aspect, the parietal lobe is separated from the occipital lobe by the parieto-occipital sulcus and its inferior continuation, the calcarine fissure. This region of the parietal lobe is subdivided into two major structures, the anterior positioned posterior paracentral lobule (a continuation of the postcentral gyrus) and the posteriorly situated precuneus. The temporal cortex lies directly under the lateral fissure. The occipital lobe is the most posterior portion of the cerebral cortex and, interestingly, is not marked by any of the major cortical fissures.

Figures 57 and 58 show the respective BA in the left hemisphere, in a saggital view of the brain.

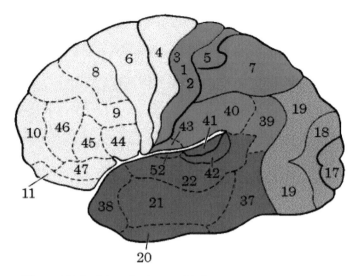

Figure 57: Left hemisphere with Brodmann areas

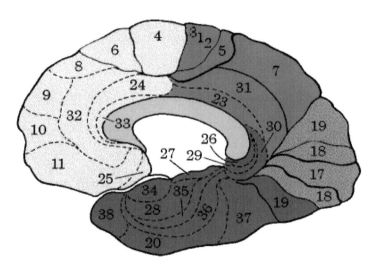

Figure 58: Sagittal view with Brodmann areas

In the following sections, I will cover the BA and generalized functions of regions thought to be associated with particular psychopathologies and normal cognitive functions. Although it is suggested that surface EEG recordings can access a maximal number of neurons, it is important to note that neurons are extremely complex and each may have connections with other regions that simply may not be traced. An example would be from Chapter 3, in which the posterior corpus callosum is reduced in volume relative to lesions in the parietal lobes. This is an extremely important consideration when evaluating the EEG and localizing the sources. We certainly may have to revisit older notions as technology advances. Additionally, I will cover specific details as determined by neuroimaging data. Although it might be advantageous to describe the areas by lobe, I will address each by the order of numerical appearance. BA 1, 2, and 3 represent the primary somatosensory cortex (PSC) located on the postcentral gyrus in the parietal lobe. BA 3 of the PSC is divided into subdivisions 3a and 3b. Each of these regions receives and projects specialized connections to thalamic nuclei. Area 3b represents the neurology of the bodily parts (e.g., homunculus) in which the size of the area corresponds to the density of sensory innervations of each bodily area. Area 3a receives input from mechanoreceptors located in muscle tissue while 3b and 1 receive input from cutaneous mechanoreceptors (Iannetti et al., 2003). Area 2 receives inputs from joints and other deep tissues. The somatosensory cortex is associated with numerous human perceptions, including temperature, chemical, and proprioception in addition to nociception and pain processes (Kirimoto et al., 2010; McCaslin, Chen, Radosevich, Cauli, & Hillman, 2010; Straube & Miltner, 2011; Zhang, Jiao, & Sun, 2011). BA 4 is the primary motor cortex in the posterior portion of the frontal lobe (Hanakawa et al., 2002; Kim et al., 2009; Kurth et al., 1998).

The motor cortex is proposed in a most logical sense to be responsible for the organization, programming, and execution of voluntary motor activity, and it is considered the main source of information for performed movements and actions (Luria, 1966). BA 5 is a somatosensory association cortex with connections to other somatosensory regions and motor areas. This region has also been shown to play a role in hand and arm movements and manipulation of objects in non-human primates (Cohen, Prud'homme, & Kalaska, 1994). BA 4 and BA 6, the premotor cortex, have extensive connections with subcortical and thalamic structures as well as sensory cortical areas and as such represent a critical mass of the cerebrum dedicated to the movement and integrative functions of the organism (Luria, 1966). BA 7 (Precuneus) is a somatosensory association cortex (Castellanos et al., 2008; Cavanna & Trimble, 2006) and is considered to be one of the more difficult regions in the cortex to functionally map, given its widespread connections and somewhat protected orientation within the brain (Cavanna & Trimble, 2006). Although the precuneus and posterior cingulate are often grouped as one locale in the default network of the brain (discussed later in this section), there are clear cytoarchitectural differences in the posterior cingulate transition from isocortex to limbic cortex (Cavanna & Trimble, 2006).

Compared to primates, the precuneus encompasses a larger, and more developed mass of volume in human beings. Most notably, it has the most complex columnar cortical organization and is among the last regions to myelinate (Cavanna & Trimble, 2006). It is also shown to be involved in a wide range of higher order cognitive functions, including attention, self-referential and self-recognition tasks, theory of mind, working memory, and numerous other cognitive processes. As shown in the examples of parietal dysfunction in earlier chapters, the precuneus is a target of more sophisticated neurofeedback techniques.

The precuneus shares connections with medial and lateral parietal, dorsolateral prefrontal, frontal, anterior cingulate, and superior temporal cortices. It also has extensive subcortical connections, including the thalamus, striatum, claustrum, and brain-stem (zona incerta, superior colliculus, dorsolateral pontine nucleus, and pregeniculate nucleus to name a few) (Cavanna & Trimble, 2006). The posterior parietal cortex (areas 5 and 7) has long been known to be concerned with the perception of tactile objects, body form and extrapersonal space (Chow & Hutt, 1953). This has been demonstrated by ablation experiments in monkeys and by clinical studies of the 'parietal lobe syndrome' (Bolton & Calhoun, 1971; Chakravorty, 1982; Matousek, Brunovsky, Edman, & Wallin, 2001; Money, 1973; Ramachandran, 1995). However, much of the cytoarchitecture of the precuneus is based on non-human primates that have underdeveloped posteriomedial parietal areas as compared to humans (Cavanna & Trimble, 2006). Certain aspects of these functions relate to vision as well as to somesthesia. The location and extent of lesions are difficult to specify precisely in both ablation experiments and in humans with brain injury site of higher-order cognitive processing, somatosensory processing, and possibly motivational and emotional processes, given their extensive connections and associations with self-relative processes.

BA 8 in the frontal lobe includes the frontal eye fields and plays an intricate role in self-regulation, executive attention, and self-monitoring. BA8 is active during tasks of decision-making and uncertainty (Volz, Schubotz, & von Cramon, 2005) and plays an important role in executive attention and self-regulation (Cannon, Congedo, Lubar, & Hutchens, 2009; Cannon et al., 2007; Cannon, Sokhadze, Lubar, & Baldwin, 2008), emotion (Damasio et al., 2000), and self-image processing (Butcher, 2001). BA 9 consists of the dorsolateral prefrontal cortices and is involved in various functions, including working memory, rare stimuli, affect, arithmetic, as well as in attention (Brazdil et al., 2007; Jahanshahi, Dirnberger, Fuller, & Frith, 2000; MacDonald, Cohen, Stenger, & Carter, 2000; Seidman et al., 2006). BA 10 is the most rostral portion of the superior and middle frontal gyri and is active in emotion and physiological response to external stimuli (Critchley, Daly, et al., 2000; Critchley, Elliott, Mathias, & Dolan, 2000).

Evidence from human studies on the role of PFC in cortisol regulation stems largely from functional neuroimaging studies investigating neural correlates of psychological stress processing. Functional neuroimaging studies on, for example, language, perception, navigation, and motor control (Ramnani & Miall, 2004; Ramnani & Owen, 2004) and studies with affect regulation components (Davidson, 2004; Levesque, Joanette, et al., 2003; Levesque et al., 2004), show that activation patterns in area 10 can occur during virtually any kind of cognitive paradigm, from the simplest conditioning paradigms to the most complex tests involving memory, judgment, or problem-solving. Lesions to this region in humans do not impair performance on tests of intellectual performance, memory, language, motor skills, visual perception, and problem-solving abilities. Instead, specific impairments occur in self-organized behavior or open-ended procedures that require the individual to monitor and regulate self in an organized manner and in tasks that require self-maintenance of attentional processes, which may also be placed under the category of self-regulation (Burgess, Dumontheil, & Gilbert, 2007).

Recent PET data investigated psychosocial stress and the results showed that increased cortisol correlated significantly with increased BGM in medial prefrontal cortices BA9 and BA10 (Kern et al., 2008). However, findings that are more salient were associated with increased BGM in lateral aspects of the prefrontal cortex, which is consistent with findings showing that unpleasant emotions, including anxiety, tend to show patterns of increased right prefrontal activity (Davidson, 2002; Davidson, Coe, Dolski, & Donzella, 1999). Similar data propose that the prefrontal cortex provides a top-down mechanism for regulation of the HPA response with consideration given to the region and nature of the stressor. Moreover, regions in left prefrontal (BA6, BA9) have been shown to be inversely correlated with increased amygdala activity (Dedovic et al., 2009). Perfusion fMRI data showed increased activity in right hemisphere regions as a result of psychological stress while cortisol showed positive associations with increased activity in the anterior cingulate, putamen, posterior cingulate, precuneus, and insular cortex (Wang et al., 2005). The dorsolateral prefrontal cortices (DLPFC) have been shown to be active in a high degree of cognitive, attention and memory related experiments (Barde & Thompson-Schill, 2002; Dehaene & Changeux, 2000; Fuster, 2000a, 2000b). Specifically regions in the left prefrontal cortex have been shown to be involved in working memory, disinhibition, and cognitive processes. The left PFC is considered involved in attention and conceptualization processes. Additionally, it is involved in theory of mind tasks, interpreting the mental states of others and self and other facial recognition (Brady, Campbell, & Flaherty, 2004; Cannon, Congedo, Lubar, & Hutchens, 2009; Cannon et al., 2007; Cannon & Lubar, 2008; Cannon, Lubar, Gerke, Thornton, Hutchens, & McCammon, 2006; DeBruine, 2004; Gara et al., 1993).

Studies have shown that mental state considerations that explicitly reflect on aspects of one's own mental state or attributions made about the mental states of others (e.g., theory of mind tasks) employ these dorsal anterior cingulate and dorsal medial prefrontal regions (Frith & Frith, 2006; Gusnard, Akbudak, Shulman, & Raichle, 2001; Gusnard, 2005). Similarly, imaging studies targeting retrieval of personal or episodic memories involving verbal and nonverbal material (Cabeza & Nyberg, 2000; Cabeza et al., 2003) have implicated the same prefrontal region in working memory tasks. Deficits in left prefrontal and occipital regions have been shown to lead to disruptions of self-monitoring and self-evaluation processes that also involve limbic and brainstem fear centers (Lidell, Brown, et al., 2005). Studies have demonstrated that depressed individuals had decreased left anterior activation characterized by increased alpha activity compared with individuals not experiencing depression. Lesions to the left hemisphere have been shown to produce increased depression, dysthymia, and negative emotions associated with dysphoric mood. Interestingly, lesions to the right hemisphere, in prefrontal regions have been associated with dysfunction in interpreting the emotional states of others as well as deficits in social appropriateness and intrapersonal monitoring (Lubar et al., 2003).

BA 11 and 12 along with BA 25 subgenual cingulate make up the orbitofrontal cortex and contain the orbital and rectal gyri. Area 12 is orbital-medial prefrontal region of the frontal lobe. Inclusively, the orbitofrontal cortex (OFC) is instrumental to emotional regulation, encoding and retrieval, self-regulation, and most cognitive processes in normal populations. It is also implicated in numerous psychological disorders, including schizophrenia (Lacerda et al., 2007; Toro, Hallak, Dunham, & Deakin, 2006), depression, obsessive-compulsive and anxiety disorders (Drevets, 2007; Toro & Deakin, 2005), personality disorders (New et al., 2007; Resnick, Driscoll, & Lamar, 2007), and substance use disorders (Goldstein, Tomasi, et al., 2007). Along with other regions included in this review, it is also involved in tasks regarding social cognition, interpreting the mental states of others (theory of mind), self-reference, encoding, reality monitoring, suicidal ideation, and empathic processes (Berthoz, Armony, Blair, & Dolan, 2002; Critchley, 2005; du Boisgueheneuc et al., 2006; Fleck, Daselaar, Dobbins, & Cabeza, 2006; Goel et al., 1995; Kensinger & Schacter, 2005; Kim & Hamann, 2007; Walton, Croxson, Behrens, Kennerley, & Rushworth, 2007). The OFC is one of the more metabolically active regions in the default network of the brain. It shows increased activity during the processing of self and self-relatedness as well as theory of mind tasks (assigning mental states to others), plays a particular role in negative self-perception, and an important role in the development of addictive disorders. Its location in the brain and connections to neocortex, thalamus, limbic structures, and brain stem nuclei implicate it in a wide range of human behaviors and psychological dysfunctions (Gusnard, 2005; Gusnard et al., 2001; Nelson et al., 2009).

Cortical regions, including the amygdale, that share reciprocal connections with the OFC have shown visceral effects when stimulated. These OFC/amygdala connections may also relay and maintain visceral information about the state of the organism. Levesque et al. (2003) demonstrated that BOLD signal differences were significantly higher during sadness than in a suppression condition. Bilateral regional activations associated with sadness occurred in anterior temporal pole (BA 21 and BA 38) and the midbrain, as well as in the right ventrolateral prefrontal cortex (VLPFC) (BA 47), left amygdala, and left insula. In the suppression condition, significant activation was noted in the right OFC (BA 11) and right LPFC (BA 9). Additionally, positive correlations between self-report ratings of sadness and blood oxygenation level dependent (BOLD) signal increases in the right OFC (BA 11) and right LPFC (BA 9). Thus, area 11 in conjunction with other regions may play an important role in self-affect regulation, evaluative processing, and self-monitoring of internal states (Levesque et al., 2003). Data on emotional processes suggest a common neural network involving the prefrontal cortex, particularly BA 9 and 10, amygdala, insula, basal ganglia, and anterior cingulate. In particular, negative affect generally elicits activation in the right prefrontal cortex (RPFC), amygdala, and insula, whereas the left prefrontal cortex is associated with positive emotion and appetitive goals along with reward-related cortical regions (Davidson & Irwin, 1999; Davidson, Irwin, Anderle, & Kalin, 2003; Hejmadi, Davidson, & Rozin, 2000; Salomons, Johnstone, Backonja, & Davidson, 2004; van Reekum et al., 2007; Wang et al., 2005).

BA 13 is the insular cortex. The insular cortex plays an active role in choices made from an affective rather than cognitive perspective. The insular cortex is a region of convergence of multisensory inputs implicated in numerous human functions (Craig, 2009b). Recent data demonstrated that the insula in conjunction with the thalamus plays an important role in activation or suspension of the default mode state as well as in epeliptiform activity (Gotman et al., 2005). It is thought to play an important role in emotion, especially the affective component of pain processing, as well as language processes (Sawamoto et al., 2000). Additionally, it plays an important role in depression relative to the default network, that is, connectivity and regional activity in the default network in depressed patients differ from controls during an emotional performance task. Importantly, regions within the default network have been significantly correlated with both depression severity and feelings of hopelessness (Sheline et al., 2009). Similar research implicates the right fronto-insular cortex in switching between central executive and default mode regions during attentional tasks (Sridharan et al., 2008).

Research has demonstrated increased levels of activity during emotion-related tasks in the amygdala, insula, and anterior cingulate cortices, with these regions being significant predictors of heart rate responses to the presentation of emotional facial expressions (Yang et al., 2007). Recent functional connectivity data, as a result of spatial specific neurofeedback training in the right AC, suggest that the right amygdala and insula exhibit significant functional connectivity (partial correlations) across all EEG frequencies (Cannon, Sokhadze, Lubar, & Baldwin, 2008). Critchley and colleagues measured simultaneous electrocardiography and brain activity during performance of cognitive and motor tasks. The results showed that activity in the dorsal anterior cingulate cortex (AC) played a role in the mediation of bodily arousal states (sympathetic activity) during the experimental tasks (Critchley et al., 2003). Synchronous functional MRI and heart rate data found that greater activation in the amygdala, anterior cingulate, and the right middle frontal gyrus predicted greater cardiac contractility during a stimulus paired with threat rather than safety (Dalton, Kalin, Grist, & Davidson, 2005). Another study assessed correlations between heart rate and fMRI BOLD signal during compassion meditation, revealing that changes in HR across states were positively associated with the right middle insula, somatosensory regions, right inferior parietal cortex, premotor regions (BA6), and the right temporal parietal junction. Notably, activation specific to the left hemisphere was more pronounced in experts than in novices (Lutz et al., 2009). Previous findings have reported similar patterns when participants perceived empathic pain from a somatosensory context (e.g., while looking at bodies in painful situations) (Danziger et al., 2009; Lamm et al., 2007).

In a recent study on the regulation of negative emotions, participants watching negative emotional stimuli showed increased activity in prefrontal regions associated with cognitive control, and this increase was suggested to be directly related to a decrease in right amygdala and insula (Lutz et al., 2009). These findings support the results of prior studies reporting that cognitive reappraisal down-regulated amygdala and insula responses to negative emotional stimuli such that the reappraisal of the negative stimuli also enhanced activity in medial, dorsolateral, and ventrolateral PFC regions previously identified in cognitive regulation of negative emotion (Egloff, Schmukle, Burns, & Schwerdtfeger, 2006; Liberzon, Phan, Decker, & Taylor, 2003; Liverant, Brown, Barlow, & Roemer, 2008; Phan et al., 2005). Research exploring the emotion of disgust reported similar regional activation in the right insular cortex and suggested that this region, in association with medial frontal and limbic regions, is directly involved in the experience of disgust (Calder, 2003). Disgust is usually described as a basic emotion that elicits avoidance behavior (Rozin & Fallon, 1987) or as a marked aversion aroused by something highly distasteful, according to traditional definition. Triggers of disgust are variable (or subjective). For example, it has been suggested that disgust response specific to food rejection is innate. A culturally relevant category of disgust stimuli includes body products, certain small animals, poor hygiene, injury, and death (Rozin & Fallon, 1987; Schienle, Schafer, Stark, Walter, & Vaitl, 2005a, 2005c).

There is disagreement about the neural substrates of disgust, especially concerning the specific role of the insular cortex, since the insular cortex activation is not restricted only to a disgust condition, it also increases in a fear condition (Schienle, Schafer, Stark, Walter, & Vaitl, 2005b). In these experiments, like those assessing self-in-experience and mental decoding tasks (Cannon et al., 2008), activation as a function of disgust and a negative view of self showed increased activation of the right amygdala, orbitofrontal, and medial prefrontal cortex, as well as the hippocampus and insular cortex. These potential neuronal assemblies are proposed to involve functionally connected neural networks, which are involved in the evaluation of ongoing stimulation with regard to the reinforcement value, maintenance of the self, and the selection of appropriate behaviors (Cannon et al., 2008; Rolls, Critchley, Browning, Hernadi, & Lenard, 1999). BA 14 and 15 have been designated in the primate cortex but have no human equivalent. BA 16 is located within the insular cortex and is not differentiated in data from neuroimaging experiments or standardized maps. BA 17 is the primary visual cortex, 18 is secondary visual cortex, and 19 is an associative visual region.

The cuneus and Brodmann Area (BA) 19 are regions of the cortex considered important to tertiary visual processes in conjunction with BA 18. BA 19 has been shown active during confrontation naming tasks (Abrahams et al., 2003) and decreased when subjects made decisions about favorite brands of consumer goods (Deppe et al., 2005). This occipital region is active during unimodal visual motion stimulation (Deutschlander et al., 2002), stereodepth perceptions (Fortin et al., 2002), "theory of mind" tasks (Goel et al., 1995), and memory retrieval (Osipova et al., 2006). BA 20 is part of the inferior lateral temporal lobe and in association with BA 37, 38, ventromedial prefrontal cortex, and limbic regions, it plays a role in higher order visual processing, recognition memory, and semantic memory (Mummery et al., 2000; Staiman, 1998). This area is also highly involved in self-recognition and self-reference and may play an important role in emotion and self-regulation (Cannon et al., 2008; Kelley et al., 2002; Kircher & Leube, 2003; Kircher, Seiferth, Plewnia, Baar, & Schwabe, 2007). BA 21 and 22 are part of the temporal cortex and play an important role in auditory and language processing; additionally, these regions are active during decision-making and other executive functions, which may emphasize their role in language and all cognitive processes (Kelley et al., 1998; Nyberg, McIntosh, Houle, Nilsson, & Tulving, 1996; Paulus, Feinstein, Leland, & Simmons, 2005). BA 23 is the ventral posterior cingulate. Posterior cingulate cortex begins at the transition from BA 24 to 23 and includes the isocortex of areas 23 and 31.

The posterior cingulate cortex (PCC) encompasses the retrosplenial cortex, which comprises area 29. The demarcation between area 30 of the retrosplenial cortex and the adjacent area 23 of the posterior cingulate isocortex on the convexity of the cingulate gyrus in the human brain has not been delineated clearly. However, several studies have demonstrated activation of 23, 29, and anterior portions during emotion and episodic memory processes. Precise functional activations are unavailable for many of the regions in the PCC (Maddock, 1999). BA 26 is the ectosplenial area (retrosplenial region). BA 28 is the entorhinal cortex (including the uncinate gyrus). Area 29 is the retrosplenial cingulate cortex. The perirhinal cortex BA 35/36 is located in the anterior and medial part of the ventral aspect of the temporal lobe.

The entorhinal cortex in turn serves as the source of the perforant pathway into the hippocampus (Buckley, 2005; Maddock, 1999). Interestingly, lesions to the perirhinal and entorhinal regions produce deficits nearly as severe as lesions to the amygdala or hippocampus, with perirhinal showing the largest degree of deficit. This suggests a very important role of these regions in self-regulation, motivation, and emotional processes (Buckley, 2005; Maddock, 1999). The entorhinal cortex provides major cortical input to the hippocampus through the perforant pathway (Zola-Morgan & Squire, 1985; Zola-Morgan, Squire, & Amaral, 1986; Zola-Morgan, Squire, Amaral, & Suzuki, 1989; Zola-Morgan, Squire, Rempel, Clower, & Amaral, 1992). It is one of the first anatomical regions to show Alzheimer disease pathology (Braak & Braak, 1985), with more than half of adults between 56 and 60 years of age having neurofibrillary tangles in at least the entorhinal region of the brain. BA 35, 36, and 28 are important in emotion, learning, memory, and other important sensory and motivational processes. BA 30 is transitional region between the posterior cingulate gyrus and the medial temporal lobe, and it is a cortical component of the limbic system. BA 31 is a dorsal part of posterior cingulate (Maddock, 1999).

The posterior cingulate (PC)/precuneus module is the only node in the default network to interact with all other nodes (Fransson & Marrelec, 2008); however, the EEG activity involved in these intrinsic interactions is not known. Similarly, research has demonstrated decreased coherency between default network regions in Alzheimer's disease, especially concerning the role of the PC and left hippocampus (Greicius, Srivastava, Reiss, & Menon, 2004). The PC is among the most metabolically active regions in the RSN in healthy individuals (Raichle et al., 2001). Moreover, diffusion tensor imaging research suggests that disruptions in functional connectivity between the PC and hippocampus produce effects in connections to the medial temporal and frontal cortices (Zhou et al., 2008). Thus, PC plays an important role in memory as well as verbal and integrative functionality (Lustig et al., 2003).

The PC (BA 31) is a vaulted structure located bilaterally along the mid-line. It is dorsal to the corpus callosum, inferior to the cingulate sulcus, and superior to the callosal sulcus (Vogt, Nimchinsky, Vogt, & Hof, 1995). The PC is adjacent to the AC, such that the AC and PC, inclusively with central cingulate (CG), form the cingulate gyrus. Functionally, the PC is considered an evaluative region, involved in assessing environmental stimuli and memory functions (Vogt, Finch, & Olson, 1992) and pain (Vogt, Derbyshire, & Jones, 1996). It is also considered important for verbal production and comprehension in addition to attentional processes and higher order visual processing (Cannon et al., 2009; Choo et al., 2008).

BA 27 is the piriform cortex associated primarily with olfaction in non-human primates. The exact function in humans is not known. One of the primary brain regions involved in consciousness, self-awareness, learning, reward, and decision-making processes is the anterior cingulate gyrus (AC) (Devinsky, Morrell, & Vogt, 1995). It consists of Brodmann Areas 24, 32, 33, and 25. The pathology of major psychiatric disorders is yet to be fully understood. However, structural and functional neuroimaging studies along with postmortem investigations have provided some indications as to which cortical regions may be predominantly affected in these disorders. One such candidate brain region is the anterior cingulate cortex. Functional imaging studies have revealed altered blood flow and/or glucose metabolism in this region in patients diagnosed with schizophrenia (Buchsbaum et al., 2007; Buchsbaum et al., 2009; Buchsbaum et al., 2006; Friston, Liddle, Frith, Hirsch, & Frackowiak, 1992; Frith, Friston, Liddle, & Frackowiak, 1992; Hazlett et al., 2008; Jansen, Hegde, & Boutros, 2004; Liddle, 1992; Liddle, Friston, Frith, & Frackowiak, 1992; Pascual-Marqui et al., 1999; Tislerova et al., 2008), major depressive disorder (Bench et al., 1992; Bjork et al., 2008; Fingelkurts, Rytsala, Suominen, Isometsa, & Kahkonen, 2006, 2007; Pizzagalli et al., 2001; Pizzagalli, Bogdan, Ratner, & Jahn, 2007; Pizzagalli, Nitschke, et al., 2002; Pollock & Schneider, 1990), and bipolar disorder (Cook, Shukla, & Hoff, 1986; Dewan, Haldipur, Boucher, Ramachandran, & Major, 1988; Pizzagalli, Goetz, Ostacher, Iosifescu, & Perlis, 2008) compared to healthy controls. Similarly, structural imaging studies have reported reduced grey matter volumes in the anterior cingulate cortex in these disorders (Ballmaier et al., 2004). Further evidence implicating the anterior cingulate cortex in major psychiatric disorders comes from postmortem studies, which have revealed a number of histological and neurochemical abnormalities within this region. Cell counting studies have identified a reduction in neuronal size along with lower glial cell densities in SCZ, BPD, and MDD. Evidence also suggests abnormalities of the GABAergic and glutamatergic systems. Indeed, reduced density of GABAergic interneurons has been described in this brain region in each of these disorders. Furthermore, reductions in synaptic markers have also been observed within the anterior cingulate cortex in both SCZ and mood disorders (Beasley et al., 2006; Chana, Landau, Beasley, Everall, & Cotter, 2003; Cotter et al., 2002).

Animal studies showed that the AC is intricately involved in the encoding and schemata formation (neural pathways) of the external and internal worlds. Helmeke and colleagues studied social and environmental influence on infant rats with: (i) undisturbed control animals, (ii) handled animals, (iii) animals repeatedly deprived from their parents during the first 3 postnatal weeks, and (iv) animals treated similar to group (iii) and thereafter kept in chronic social isolation. The results of this and a parallel study revealed the sensitivity of the dorsal AC to environmental changes and emotional challenges during early periods of postnatal brain development. Experience-induced synaptic alterations were observed several weeks after the animals were returned to undisturbed social conditions, indicating that these environmentally induced arborization processes can be enduring and perhaps even permanent. The observed elevated, presumably excitatory, synaptic input into a cortical part of the limbic system may reflect developmental adaptations of the maturing brain to repeated emotional challenges (Helmeke, Ovtscharoff, Poeggel, & Braun, 2001; Helmeke, Poeggel, & Braun, 2001; Ovtscharoff, Helmeke, & Braun, 2006).

The AC has one of the highest densities of opioid receptors in the central nervous system and plays an intricate role in nociception, monitoring of the affective component in pain processing, as well as substance abuse disorders. Studies have demonstrated that lesions or removal of specific portions of the AC affected the experience of pain, specifically, reducing the affective component and the experience of painful stimuli. Morphine injections elevate cerebral blood flow to rostral and ventral portions of AC. Additionally, the AC projects extensive afferent thalamocortical connections involved with enkephalin-immunoreactive neurons and noradrenergic neurons in addition to opioid neurons in locus cereleus. These projections and functions implicate the AC in numerous clinical syndromes (Nimchinsky, Vogt, Morrison, & Hof, 1995; Oya et al., 2005; Vogt, Wiley, & Jensen, 1995; Woodward, Chang, Janak, Azarov, & Anstrom, 1999). Research indicates that persons with attention deficit/hyperactivity disorder (ADHD) fail to activate the cognitive division of the AC during Stroop interference tasks. Similarly, persons with ADHD produce slower reaction times to stimuli and this involves response selection processes in the AC (Colla et al., 2008). Studies suggest that the cognitive division of the AC is activated during divided attention tasks, and the activation of affective division is decreased during cognitive tasks and vice versa (Bush et al., 2000; Devinsky et al., 1995).

PET and fMRI experiments have reported activation of the AC in memory (Dudukovic & Wagner, 2007; Kaneda & Osaka, 2008; Nyberg et al., 2003), cognition (Allman, Hakeem, Erwin, Nimchinsky, & Hof, 2001), emotion (Allman et al., 2001; Beauregard, Levesque, & Bourgouin, 2001; Bush et al., 2000; Phan, Liberzon, Welsh, Britton, & Taylor, 2003; Phan, Wager, Taylor, & Liberzon, 2002), as well as decision-making and reward processes (Bush et al., 2002; Kennerley, Walton, Behrens, Buckley, & Rushworth, 2006; Walton et al., 2007). Similar epilepsy and lesion studies indicated that the AC plays a direct role in visceromotor functions, control of vocalization, and communication of internal states, skeletomotor control, nociception, and memory processes, as well as language and working memory/attentive processes. It is also implicated in social interactions, affect-regulation, and psychopathology (Bush et al., 2000; Devinsky et al., 1995). Several theories relating to the role of the AC in attentional and executive processes have been suggested, without clarifying the interactions between the AC and the left and right dorsolateral prefrontal cortices (LPFC and RPFC), even though attentional processes are the most investigated function of the AC (Bench et al., 1993; Posner & Rothbart, 1998).

It has been proposed that the AC detects the need for executive control and signals the prefrontal cortex (PFC) to execute the control (Cohen, Botvinik, & Carter, 2000; Markela-Lerenc et al., 2004). Similarly, research proposed that the AC is in effect a gating mechanism between the cortex and subcortical regions (Pizzagalli et al., 2003). Area 33 is part of the anterior cingulate dorsal of the corpus callosum. Evaluation of stimuli and decision-making processes (i.e., executive functions) involves numerous brain regions, including those implicated in the much debated brain reward system (BRS) (Woodward et al., 1999). The brain reward system (BRS) is proposed to involve mesolimbic, prefrontal, and basal ganglia structures, including the insular, somatosensory, orbitofrontal (OFC), anterior cingulate (AC), and dorsolateral prefrontal cortices (DLPFC), as well as the amygdala, hippocampus, midline thalamic nuclei, ventral pallidus, pedunculopontine nucleus, hypothalamus, substantia nigra, and ventral tegmental area (VTA). Additionally, these regions are implicated in a specific reward network involving the nucleus accumbens (NaC) that is affected by drug and alcohol abuse, gambling, and most appetitive behaviors. The NaC is a primary source of inhibitory GABAergic neurotransmitters (Bechara, 2005; Everitt & Robbins, 2005). This reward system is active during the comprehension of humor, which is also suggested to involve equivalent faculties as social communication and social processing (Brown, Paul, Symington, & Dietrich, 2005).

The neurofeedback and self-regulation disciplines as well as neuroimaging experiments need to clarify **Reward** and **Reinforcement** for two explicit reasons. First, in many situations in the human condition, the rules describing interdependencies between different actions do exist and exploitation of these rules can lead to one type of reward being more salient compared to another. Secondly, abstract concepts involve rules governing rewarding behaviors and in the most basic sense, appreciation of the abstraction invariably depends on a congruency effect of both language and cognition on reward learning and decision-making. These types of reward processes are shown to involve dorsal and ventral striatum and ventromedial prefrontal cortex (O'Doherty, Hampton, & Kim, 2007; Schonberg, Daw, Joel, & O'Doherty, 2007). Functional magnetic resonance imaging (fMRI) investigations of brain regions implicated in humor have increased in the past few years, and many of these studies utilize methods in which the participants rated cartoons, television clips or written words, jokes, and humorous stories. Much of the research reported similar results, with increased activation of the left temporo-occipital junction, left inferior frontal gyrus, supplementary motor area (BA 6), and a subcortical network involving the ventral striatum, Nucleus Accumbens (NaC), and other hypothalamic and amygdaloid regions (Mobbs, Greicius, Abdel-Azim, Menon, & Reiss, 2003; Moran, Wig, Adams, Janata, & Kelley, 2004).

Compared to left frontal damage, damage to the right frontal cortex (aphasics) negatively influences performance on nonverbal cartoon completion tasks, with diminished capacity to establish clarity without impairment to the sensitivity and appreciation of the surprise element (Bihrle, Brownell, Powelson, & Gardner, 1986). Studies have identified greater bilateral activation of AC, left middle frontal gyrus, right posterior cingulate, the left parietal lobe, bilateral caudate, and left parahippocampal gyrus in encoding experiments during correct expected outcomes (Kosson et al., 2006). Duncan and Owen (2000) explored the role of PFC in response to conflict, task novelty, and a number of elements in working memory, working-memory delay, and perceptual difficulty, and found plausible joint influence of three PFC regions: mid-dorsolateral PFC, mid-ventrolateral PFC, and the dorsal anterior cingulate cortex. These regions were posited to form a general network recruited by diverse challenges, such as response selection, working memory maintenance, and stimulus recognition. The DLPFC has been implicated as a key substrate mediating various executive functions, including representation of task demand, working memory (Levy & Goldman-Rakic, 2000), response selection (Rowe et al., 2000), and response switching (Garavan et al., 2002). The AC is proposed to be preferentially activated by competing information streams (Hester et al., 2004) in order to regulate and control executive functions.

BA 37 is the fusiform gyrus. PET and electrophysiological measurements have designated posterior inferior temporal cortex (BA 37) as important for object naming and visual object recognition memory (Haxby et al., 2001; Nakamura, Honda, et al., 2000; Nakamura, Kawashima, et al., 2000; Tanaka, 1997). BA 38 is a temporal lobe region, more notably described as the temporal pole - the most rostral part of superior and middle temporal gyri. The temporal pole is of course more prone to damage due to the spiny bones in the skull. It is associated with social and emotion processes and decision-making and has extensive connections with the amygdala and orbital frontal cortex (Dupont, 2002). BA 39 is the angular gyrus situated at the interface between the posterior parietal and occipital lobes. BA39 is thought to be involved in the integration of visual and tactile stimuli in addition to speech. Lesions to this area result in dyslexia or alexia plus agraphia (Damasio & Geschwind, 1984). BA 40 is the post central gyrus (portions of the supramarginal gyrus). BA 40 is involved in the integration of visual and tactile information, in addition to attentional processes (e.g., somatosensory, language, self-regulation). The AC and BA 40 have been shown to have an intricate relationship to sustained attention tasks in addition to cognitive and affective processing (Cabeza & Nyberg, 2000; Cannon et al., 2009; Cannon et al., 2007; De Ridder, Van Laere, Dupont, Menovsky, & Van de Heyning, 2007). BA 41 is in the superior aspect of the temporal lobe (located in a series of transverse gyri, called Heschl's gyri that form the inferior bank of the lateral fissure). This area corresponds to the primary auditory cortex. BA 42 is in the dorsal-lateral margin of the superior temporal gyrus and is associated with higher-order auditory areas that surround the primary auditory cortex, which may represent auditory association functions (Kanai, Lloyd, Bueti, & Walsh, 2011; Lutkenhoner, 2011; Pienkowski, Munguia, & Eggermont, 2011;

Schadwinkel & Gutschalk, 2011). Area 43 is in the inferior margin of the postcentral and precentral gyri where the frontal-parietal operculum merges with the insula just below the inferior termination of the central sulcus. Area 44 is a motor cortical area in the posterior part of the inferior frontal gyrus and is involved in the production of language, especially in the left hemisphere (Broca's area). BA 45 is in the inferior frontal lobe (inferior frontal gyrus) and along with area 44 plays a role in language production and verbal fluency (Amunts et al., 2004). Area 46 is in the middle frontal gyrus and anterior part of the inferior frontal gyrus (Burns & Fahy, 2010; Clerget, Winderickx, Fadiga, & Olivier, 2009; de Vries et al., 2010; Ford, McGregor, Case, Crosson, & White, 2010; Kotz et al., 2010; Pang, Wang, Malone, Kadis, & Donner, 2011; Vaden, Piquado, & Hickok, 2011). Area 47 is in the anterior-ventral part of the inferior frontal gyrus. These are the most referenced areas of human study in neuroscience literature and in neuroanatomical studies of location and proposed function. Research has also found that BA 47 and the insula play an important role in the processing of temporal coherence in music (Levitin & Menon, 2003). BA 48 is in the retrosubcular area with an unknown function, although it is a recognized part of the hippocampal formation. Areas 49, 50, and 51 in the rat have no human equivalent to date. This is only a brief look at many of the regions discussed. Certainly, a more thorough examination of scientific articles and functional connectivity between regions during tasks will certainly benefit the reader.

The amygdala, like the hippocampus, shares extensive connections with the brain stem, autonomic and higher executive regions of the brain. The amygdala is important for numerous behavioral functions, including appetite, sexual behaviors, aggression, reward, decision-making, aversion, emotion, memory, social functioning, fear responses, alerting, orienting, and learning (Alonso-Deflorida & Delgado, 1958; Chen, Tenney, Kulkarni, & King, 2007; Dardou, Datiche, & Cattarelli, 2007; Egger & Flynn, 1962; Evans et al., 2007). It is also suspected to play a role in numerous psychiatric syndromes (e.g., Alzheimer's disease, depression, anxiety, and schizophrenia) (Blair, 2007; Bremner, 2007; Caetano et al., 2007; Grillon, 2007) and addictive disorders (Adinoff, 2004; Di Chiara et al., 1999). The amygdala projects and receives connections from orbitofrontal, temporal, and hypothalamic regions. There has been some disagreement about many of these connections in humans, since they are not shown in rats or hamsters. Researchers suggest this can be attributed to species-specific connections developed over time and to the complexity of the external world, since the amygdala does share extensive projections with regions involved with all sensory modalities (de Olmos, 1972).

It is also known that stimulation effects in the amygdala are habituated to very rapidly. This region, when stimulated in humans, produces similar effects as observed in animal studies, producing primarily feelings of fear or rage (Delgado et al. 1968; Stevens et al. 1969). Alternatively, stimulation of regions in the temporal lobe produced feelings of fear but not rage (Jasper, 1954). Removal of the bilateral temporal lobes, including the amygdale, produced behavioral changes, such as a decrease in belligerence and reductions in fear to normally fear-inducing objects, tendencies to investigate orally and contact inedible objects, and increases in inappropriate sexual behaviors. These symptoms are collectively referred to as Kluever-Bucy Syndrome (1939). The amygdala, like the hippocampus and other limbic regions, plays an important role in many adaptive human behaviors in addition to dysfunctional contexts.

The hippocampus has extensive afferent and efferent connections throughout the cortex and is thought to be instrumental to a variety of human behaviors, including, memory, language, emotion, executive functions, learning, reward, decision making, mating behavior, and long-term potentiation of stress (Awad, Warren, Scott, Turkheimer, & Wise, 2007; Bast, 2007; Boutros et al., 2007). Dysfunctions in the hippocampal formation are implicated in numerous psychiatric disorders, including depression (Gass & Riva, 2007; Maletic et al., 2007; Sahay & Hen, 2007), schizophrenia (Barch, 2005; Woodruff-Pak & Gould, 2002), bipolar disorder (Frey et al., 2007; Itokawa & Yoshikawa, 2007), and addictive disorders (del Olmo et al., 2006; Nestler, 2001; Robbins & Everitt, 2002). The hippocampus is involved in memory and the processing of emotion, stress, and long-term potentiation processes of learning (Diamond, Campbell, Park, Halonen, & Zoladz, 2007; Joels, Krugers, & Karst, 2007). Research has demonstrated that the medial temporal lobes and the hippocampus are involved primarily in learning and memory as well as a in the process of autobiographical memory (AM) (Gluck & Bluck, 2007; Kirwan, Bayley, Galvan, & Squire, 2008; Nadel, Campbell, & Ryan, 2007). Regions functionally connected to the hippocampus during stimulus retrieval did not differentiate specific episodic memories from general AM retrieval, indicating that these memories share some aspects of the memory retrieval network. Similarly, Addis, Moscovitch, and colleagues (2004) reported no differences in hippocampal activation between specific and general AM retrieval, suggesting that temporal specificity, on its own, is not a key modulator of hippocampal activation. Three retrieval conditions activated a similar set of brain regions associated with autobiographical memory, including medial temporal lobe structures. Hippocampal activation did not change as a function of either multiple retrievals or the passage of time. Although the passage of time did not influence the activation of the precuneus, lateral prefrontal cortex, parietal cortex, lateral temporal lobe, and perirhinal cortex, it increased after multiple retrievals (Nadel et al., 2007). Episodic autobiographical images did not show a significant bias towards preferential retrieval from any particular life period; instead, they were retrieved from across the entire life span.

Activation in the right parietal regions, cuneus, precuneus, and left temporal regions has been associated with the generation of specific images while regions that are more specifically devoted to episodic memory retrieval and imagery are shown active during the generation of episodic autobiographical images (Gardini, Cornoldi, De Beni, & Venneri, 2006). Controlled autobiographical condition (directed memory recall) elicited greater activity in regions associated with self-referential processing (medial prefrontal cortex), visual/spatial memory (visual and parahippocampal regions), and recollection (hippocampus). The photo paradigm provides a way of investigating the functional neuroanatomy of real-life episodic memory under rigorous experimental control (Cabeza et al., 2004). Memories of experienced events contain sensory-perceptual episodic knowledge that is stored in occipital networks while memories of imagined events contain generic imagery generated from frontal networks (Conway, Pleydell-Pearce, Whitecross, & Sharpe, 2003). Of particular note, encoding deficiencies are more important than retrieval deficits in understanding the causes of episodic memory decline in older adults (Friedman, Nessler, & Johnson, 2007), and it is known that early AM are preserved in Alzheimer's disease to some extent (Sartori, Snitz, Sorcinelli, & Daum, 2004).

5.1: The Brain's Default Network: Neuro-Affective-Development and the Organization of the Self

Self-organization is a fundamental process in the developing human being. This process is formulated through interactions with the environment, including social relationships, functional relationships with objects, and an intimate relationship with self. In many situations, individuals interact with the environment based on reference to the self and its influence on internal states. A default core of self in the brain involves cortical midline and brain stem centers that are active in affective (emotional) processes and self-affect-regulation (Panksepp, 2003, 2005). Supporting evidence indicates that a core self is an adaptation that is species specific, and maintains equilibrium in the overall functioning of the species within the context of its social, cultural, and behavioral environments (Call & Tomasello, 2008; Rilling et al., 2007). It is known that critical periods in neural development exist and disruptions or delay in these specific periods can severely affect maturation and specificity of human functioning. Case studies of feral children (e.g., Genie, Kamala, & Amala) demonstrated that the absence of certain experiences early in life could not be compensated for by later exposure. More simply, the individual cannot make up for earlier lack of experiential learning and exposure (McCrone, 2002).

A more recent notion posits that the concepts of experience-expectant and experience-dependent sensitive periods can be viewed as organizing constructs that highlight the role that care giving and other environmental factors may play in the ontogenesis of neuro-regulatory and self-regulatory processes across the lifespan (Cicchetti & Rogosch, 1997). These concepts represent fundamental processes in the neuro-affective-developmental regulation of emotion that is of considerable interest concerning the effects of negative life experiences or negative percepts of self and self-in-experience on the developing human being (Cannon et al., 2008; Izard, Libero, Putnam, & Haynes, 1993).

Studies have shown differences between infants of depressed mothers and controls in the frontal EEG patterns. More specifically, there was increased frontal activity during sad expressions in frontal but not parietal regions. The authors concluded that infants of depressed mothers show greater amplitude of EEG power in right frontal cortex during the expression of negative emotions (Dawson, Panagiotides, Klinger, & Spieker, 1997). Research with 3-month old infants of depressed mothers demonstrated that the infants could discriminate sad from happy expressions but they did not perceive sad expressions as novel (Hernandez-Reif, Field, Diego, Vera, & Pickens, 2006). This is in line with adult data of depressed individuals, such that adults tend to exhibit asymmetries in frontal lobes specific to excess alpha frequency in the left prefrontal cortex. These frontal asymmetries are likely to involve brain regions associated with affect, including the anterior cingulate cortex (Devinsky et al., 1995).

A growing body of literature has demonstrated that prenatal exposure to substances of abuse may adversely influence normal development, including cognitive and affective processing (Singer et al., 2005). The likelihood of developing attentional disorders may be increased in children exposed to substances in utero (Mayes, 1999). Exposure to toxins inhibits reuptake of dopamine, norepinephrine, and serotonin in cortical regions involved in both attention and arousal. Animal studies have shown that prenatal exposure to cocaine does impair selective attention processes (Stanwood & Levitt, 2001; Stanwood, Washington, & Levitt, 2001).

Neural pathways (schemata) are formed early in the development process in order to organize our social, familial, and self-concepts. Within this context, the encoding of experiential information through learning and perception are on a developmental continuum. A combination of both internal and external worlds can produce negative effects on the developing self-concept. This self-concept, which may begin as early as 10-months of age, if influenced by negative experiences and a prevalent pattern of negative self-reference (perception), may increase an individual's likelihood to develop psychological distress (Gendolla, Abele, Andrei, Spurk, & Richter, 2005; Parker, 1994; Schafer, 1973). In essence, self-organization, self-perception, social and familial identity, and self-definition may begin to form very early in the developmental process. Additionally, early childhood activates brain regions involved in imitation, affect interpretation, and responsiveness, and in the broadest sense, perceptual processing of facial expressions and the environment, by means of mirror neuron pathways in the brain.

These mirror neurons are involved in processing external gestures, prosody, and posture. These neural pathways also play a key role in the infant's interactions with primary caregiver. Moreover, the child is able to interact, sense, imitate, and respond to the caregiver, which may in turn influence the development of a theory of mind (Jones, 2009; Learmonth, Lamberth, & Rovee-Collier, 2005; Meltzoff, 1990).

In prior works, we have provided an operational definition of experiential schemata (self-in-experience). Self-perception and experiential schemata involve a neurologic progression in human development that involves a fundamental self-organization process.

This self-organization process is based on the formulation of concepts of self that originate from the perceptions of self (endogenous) formed through interactions with others and the environment (exogenous). These encoded schemata become the foundation for prevailing emotions, motivations, attitudes, and attributions related to self and self-in-the-world, which are maintained, reinforced, and entrenched in neural coding mechanisms formed through dendritic arborization over the lifespan (Cannon et al., 2008). These perceptual processes can lead to the development of a self-perpetuating, negative-reinforcement circuit. This circuit or network is specific to negative affective processes, which in turn lead to the misinterpretation and personalization of interactions and events through an unregulated, dysfunctional dendritic pruning process. In other words, synapses are errantly pruned, i.e., disallowing the adaptation and dispensation of new information related to self and self-in-experience. In other words, the self in essence can become a negatively conditioned stimulus involving core self and default mode brain regions. Research has shown that negative self-esteem and negative self-image can have deleterious effects on social and interpersonal relationships and play a role in numerous psychological disorders, including anorexia/bulimia, social phobia, depression, anxiety, schizophrenia, and substance related disorders (Fries, Frey, & Pongratz, 1977; Gneo, Natoli, Menghini, & Galanti, 1986; Gordon, Lee, Dulcan, & Finegold, 1986).

Although genetic factors largely guide brain development, environmental factors and early experience sculpt its final form. Exposure to traumatic events, such as childhood abuse and neglect, has been associated with alterations in the size or functional activity of various brain regions (e.g., Andersen et al., 2008; Bremner et al., 1997; De Bellis et al., 1999, 2002b; De Bellis & Kuchibhatla, 2006; Richert et al., 2006; Teicher et al., 2004; Teicher et al., 1997; Tomoda et al., 2009a). Childhood maltreatment has been implicated in numerous forms of psychopathology, including depression (Gibb, Butler, & Beck, 2003; Spertus, Yehuda, Wong, Halligan, & Seremetis, 2003; Toth, Manly, & Cicchetti, 1992), anxiety (Gibb et al., 2003; Spertus et al., 2003), schizophrenia (Read, van Os,

Morrison, & Ross, 2005), posttraumatic stress (Spertus et al., 2003), and substance use disorders (Kendler et al., 2000). Childhood abuse, which may affect as many as one in five individuals in this country (McCauley et al., 1997), is one of the most common traumatic events that lead to the development of PTSD (Kessler et al., 1995). Several retrospective studies have found that individuals with bipolar disorder report a higher rate of childhood abuse than do those with unipolar depression (Hyun, Friedman, & Dunner, 2000; Levitan et al., 1998) or normal controls (Neeren, Alloy, & Abramson, 2008). In the largest study to date, approximately half of bipolar disorder patients reported a history of severe childhood abuse (Leverich et al., 2002).

Adults that had been exposed to extreme verbal abuse in childhood showed increased volume in the left superior temporal gyrus (BA 22) as contrasted with non-abused group. This region in the temporal lobe maintains connections with Wernicke's (language interpretation and creation) and Broca's areas (production and communication). Further data indicated volume reductions in the cingulum bundle volume in the LH that is thought to be involved in PTSD and limbic irritability, since it is the most prominent tract that connects the limbic system to the neocortex (cingulate gyrus) (Choi, Jeong, Rohan, Polcari, & Teicher, 2009; Teicher, 2002; Teicher, Glod, Surrey, & Swett, 1993; Teicher, Samson, Polcari, & Andersen, 2009; Teicher, Samson, Sheu, Polcari, & McGreenery, 2010). In these studies of abuse, fornix reductions have been associated with anxiety and somatic complaints. We might also consider the connections with the hippocampus and septal area and their importance in learning, novelty, and numerous processes, including emotion.

The hypothalamic-pituitary-adrenal (HPA) axis (Yehuda et al., 1995a,b,c) plays an important role in response to stress. Corticotropin-releasing factor (CRF) released during stress (Chappell et al., 1986) from nerve terminals originating in the paraventricular nucleus of the hypothalamus increases the secretion of adrenocorticotropin hormone

(ACTH) from the anterior pituitary, which in turn stimulates release of glucocorticoids from the adrenal (Arborelius et al., 1999). The hippocampus inhibits CRF release from the hypothalamus (Herman et al., 1989; Jacobson & Sapolsky, 1991). Early stress is also associated with life-long increases in sensitivity of the noradrenergic system (Bremner et al., 1996a,b; Francis et al., 1999; Sanchez et al., 2001; Vermetten & Bremner, 2002). Noradrenergic input stimulates the release of CRF from the paraventricular nucleus of the hypothalamus. Maternal separation resulted in an increased release of norepinephrine in the paraventricular nucleus of the hypothalamus.

It is also necessary to provide an operational definition that has been to some extent evasive since William James posited, "everyone knows what attention is." In the context of this work, attention is a specific, sequential cerebral directive for the reduction of sensory responses to or from competing streams of exogenous and endogenous stimuli in order to facilitate the encoding and subsequent storage of a stream or streams of interest for a selective potential or immediate best response. This operational definition includes those variants of attention discussed by other authors and researchers (e.g., focused, selective, visual, auditory, and tactile variants). Attention is inherently important and necessary to the overall executive functioning of the individual. Disruptions to attentive processes influence other cognitive processes and vice versa.

5.2: Default Network in Early Development

This section emphasizes the importance of early experiences on the default mode of brain function (Corbetta et al., 1998; Gusnard et al., 2001; Raichle et al., 2001; Raichle & Snyder, 2007; Shulman et al., 1997). The Default mode network (DMN) consists of twelve functionally related regions that consistently show increased activity compared to functionally specific cognitive tasks or eyes-opened resting conditions (Shulman et al., 1997; Shulman et al., 1999; Shulman, Schwarz, Miezin, & Petersen, 1998). The DMN is synonymous with resting state network (RSN); however, the RSN includes numerous networks of functionally connected neuronal assemblies (Damoiseaux et al., 2008; Damoiseaux et al., 2006; Fransson et al., 2007). Recent work by Fair and colleagues (2008) have demonstrated that the brain's default mode network (DMN) exhibits less functional connectivity in children compared to adults. The DMN is proposed to support such core functions as theory of mind, self-related activities, such as autobiographical self, stimulus independent thought, self-projection, self-reference, and introspective processes (Fair et al., 2008).

Another, less accepted idea is that the DMN is directly involved in self-internally directed mental activity (Gusnard et al., 2001). The reduced functional integration or synchronous activity within this default mode network in children as compared to adults stresses the importance of experience and the formation of neural pathways on the developing human being. Moreover, if this network does perform a critical role in the organization and conceptualization of self, then the effects of self-perception in relation to experiential schemata undoubtedly provide important foci for normal and abnormal development with regard to the self-organization process. A recent study demonstrated similarities in DMN structures between humans and chimpanzees, such that both species exhibited high levels of activity in rostral lateral and dorsolateral PFC. Humans showed the highest level of activity in more dorsal areas of medial prefrontal cortex (PFC) in Brodmann area (BA) 9 and BA 32, whereas chimpanzees showed more widespread activity, including activity in more ventral areas of (BA 10). Similar to human studies, higher resting state activity was shown in the posterior cingulate in chimpanzees. The left-lateralized activity related to language and concept processing or mentalizing in humans was not observed in chimpanzees (Rilling et al., 2007).

Similarly, research exploring resting state networks (RSN) in the infant brain concluded that long-range functional connectivity is evident during the earliest phases of human brain development (Fransson et al., 2007). The adult brain may include up to 10 of these RSN networks; however, five RSN were identified in the infant brain, including the medial aspects of the occipital cortex (posterior cingulate), differing from RSN attributed to predominantly cortical regions residing along the somatosensory and motor cortex in the adult brain (De Luca, Beckmann, De Stefano, Matthews, & Smith, 2006).

RSN activity in infants specific to the temporal lobe and the inferior parietal cortex that includes the primary auditory cortex in the superior temporal gyrus has also been described in the adult brain (Damoiseaux et al., 2006; De Luca et al., 2006; Greicius, Krasnow, Reiss, & Menon, 2003; White et al., 2009). Thus, we can deduce that a pattern of functional connectivity between regions in the cortex is differentially active during baseline and decreases in activity during specific tasks, considering that this pattern of resting activity or default network has been shown to be similar to some degree in chimpanzees, infants, children, and adults.

A stable, consistent pattern of neural activity and functional connectivity between neuronal assemblies within these cortical regions may provide important diagnostic considerations with respect to many developmental disorders as well as psychological syndromes in the adult population. Discovery of idiosyncratic biological markers for such disorders can only benefit our holistic understanding of psychological syndromes and enhance the development of more disorder specific treatment options and implementation of evidence based neurophysiological outcome measures.

5.3: Neuroanatomy of Default Mode Network

In the past decade, neuroimaging research has demonstrated that during specific cognitive tasks, the human brain exhibits increased spatial organization in neuronal activation (Steyn-Ross, Steyn-Ross, Wilson, & Sleigh, 2009). The default mode network (DMN) was derived from this body of neuroimaging results utilizing PET and fMRI techniques. These studies show consistent decrease in neural activity as measured by local decrease in cerebral blood flow and blood-oxygenated level-dependent (BOLD).

PET is a direct measure of local neuronal activity (Raichle, 1998), such that neural activity shows increases in regional cerebral glucose metabolism (rCGM) to brain regions involved in changing mental activities or cognitively demanding tasks (Shulman et al., 1997; Shulman et al., 1999; Shulman et al., 2001).

The fMRI BOLD response is an indirect measure of neural activity. Despite the advantages of increased spatial resolution, limitations to the temporal resolution and ambiguity associated with the interpretation and reporting of results remain (Logothetis et al., 2001; Logothetis & Wandell, 2004).

There is often a high degree of overlap in activation of brain regions during cognitive, memory, attentional, and affective tasks, which adds to the difficulty in interpreting fMRI results (Cabeza & Nyberg, 2000). Despite these challenges, this DMN effect has been replicated in numerous studies (Fransson, 2005; Gusnard et al., 2001; Raichle et al., 2001). Recent data examining self-relatedness demonstrated that the same regions often recruited during reward, including the bilateral nucleus accumbens (NaC), ventral tegmental area (VTA), and ventromedial prefrontal cortex (VMPFC), were also active during self-relatedness. Furthermore, the fMRI signal time courses showed no difference between reward and self-relatedness in early BOLD signals. Additionally, both conditions differed in late BOLD signals, with self-relatedness showing higher signal intensity. The conclusion was that sustained recruitment of the reward system is also demonstrated during self-relatedness, suggesting an important relationship between reward and self (de Greck et al., 2008).

In addition to using psychometric scales for depression, personality, attachment, and self-perception, we have utilized sLORETA to investigate the activity in the DMN during several self-related and self-specific tasks (Cannon, 2009). Figure 59 shows an example from research investigating sLORETA and the DMN during specific experimental conditions. The effect shown is similar to other neuroimaging techniques. It should be noted that not all regions in the DMN show an increase, several do not change because of differences in baseline condition. I plan to continue this line of inquiry with as many psychological assessment instruments as possible.

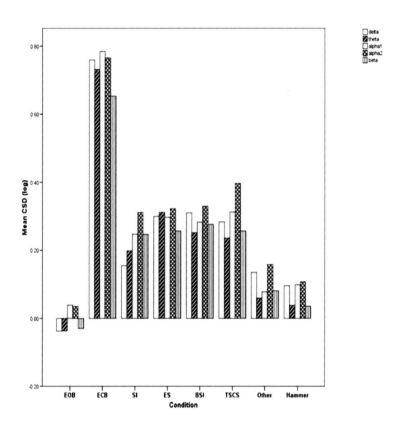

Figure 59: Grand means for current source density measured in 63 individuals (39 female and 24 male) in the default network (12 5mm³ voxels during specific experimental conditions. On the abscissa, from left to right, are the conditions: eyes-opened baseline, eyes-closed baseline, self-face, self-perception, brief symptom inventory, Tennessee self-concept scale, other face and object (hammer). On the ordinate is the current source density level. The DMN CSD between ECB and EOB shows the same effect as other neuroimaging techniques. Importantly, the DMN appears to increase preferentially relative to self and items associated with self as opposed to a picture of another face or an everyday tool.

5.4: Summary

The brain and its functions are the most challenging scientific topic. We have much to learn about the brain stem and its coordination of all human behavior, including homeostasis and its relation to the frontal lobes where our most fundamental data for operating in the world is stored. One of the most challenging concepts when using LORETA is relating the findings to other neuroimaging techniques. This is difficult for two primary reasons. First, PET and fMRI indirectly measure neural activity using different signaling techniques. Second, the EEG contains numerous subsets of data within each epoch. In considering the potential of neuromodulation, neurofeedback, and other techniques to enhance the operant behavior of the individual, this section provides important references for making hypotheses and regional data to influence decisions about intracranial sources to train. Thus far, neurofeedback techniques have been employed in the anterior cingulate, dorsolateral prefrontal cortex, precuneus, and insular cortex without report of negative effects. Psychometric scores for pre- and post- LNFB have been correlated with specific regions of interest in specific frequency domains and this data is forthcoming. The use of LORETA and qEEG in conjunction with other neuroimaging techniques can only benefit our knowledge and provide important details to aid us in understanding the functional network properties of the human brain.

CHAPTER 6

Ethical Considerations and Restrictions

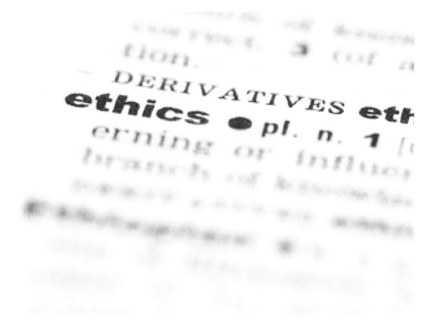

CHAPTER 6

Ethical Considerations and Restrictions

The ethical considerations in neurofeedback and functional neuroimaging are immense. The neurotherapy community inclusively adopts and adheres to the guidelines of the American Psychological Association, American Psychiatric Association, and the American Medical Association. Special circumstances should however be considered in the diagnostic procedures. It has been the policy of numerous organizations that one type of diagnostic test (or screening) is insufficient to make a definite diagnosis. In reporting the results of qEEG and LORETA to a patient, responsibility and competence should be at the forefront of this diagnostic step, such that communicating to a patient that there is evidence of a psychological disorder would have a substantial effect on all areas of the individual. Is this diagnosis-effect enhanced when the communication consists of a functional brain abnormality? This ought to be an area of intense research. Clinicians strive to provide the highest quality of service and carefully differentiate between empirically validated and experimental procedures, and those that do not, have data driven support. They hold themselves responsible for their actions and make every effort to protect their clients' welfare. Finally, they limit their services to those areas in which they have expertise and areas that exemplify the values of competence, objectivity, freedom of inquiry, and honest communication. Neuroimaging, neurofeedback, and functional network analyses are rapidly advancing fields of research, and the practitioner will do well to keep apprised of current developments. Similarly, EEG signal analysis is advancing by leaps and bounds since the beginning of this manuscript, even I am hard-pressed to keep up with its pace.

LORETA program includes explicit instructions of what would constitute a misuse and ethical violation of use. LORETA computes electric potential differences (time domain EEG/ERP) directly from scalp or from EEG cross-spectra (frequency domain). It is not for use with any other metric. Users may not attempt influence or cheat LORETA with the input. The examples of misuse occur when (1) inputting scalp electric potential spectral powers will not output LORETA (current density) spectral powers, (2) inputting scalp electric potential square roots of spectral powers will not output LORETA (current density) square roots of spectral powers, and (3) inputting scalp z-transformed-maps will not output LORETA (current density) z-transformed-values. These three invalid inputs to LORETA violate the mathematics and the physics underlying all computations. Furthermore, they violate any correct usage of statistical analysis (Frei et al., 2001; Pascual-Marqui, 1999) http://www.uzh.ch/keyinst/NewLORETA/Misuse/Misuse.htm).

6.1: Summary

The first duty charged to, and accepted by health care professions, is to first, do no harm. This entails treating the patient with the utmost confidence, respect and consideration, and utilizing evidence driven standards of care. Communicating to a patient the potential of any abnormality in the brain or its connectivities may exact deleterious effects on the patient and as such this communication should be undertaken with special attention to wording and potential damage. It is imperative to adhere to the respective guidelines and standards of practice when using qEEG and LORETA. Additionally, ethical guidelines regarding research and appropriate use of the LORETA software packages are posted and easily accessible for clarity and responsible use. It is my personal choice to treat each patient as a research participant, providing informed consent, potential side-effects, risk assessment and interventions as well as evidence of change, including statistical differences in the changes in topographical EEG, connectivities and current source density in addition to neuropsychological pre and post contrasts. The fields of neurotherapy and neuroscience are advancing at exponential rates and our ethical standards should advance likewise.

CHAPTER 7

Conclusions and Speculative Neurological/Psychological Musings

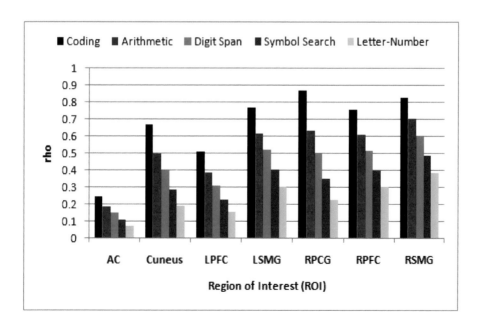

CHAPTER 7

Conclusions and Speculative Neurological/Psychological Musings

In numerous contexts, the study of the brain and its enigmatic properties can invoke much distress and confusion. I often consider how interesting it is that this organ seeks to understand itself! One of the more important concepts to develop in recent years is experience-dependent neuroplasticity. Intuitively, this has made sense to me for some time; however, empirical data demonstrating it in humans was somewhat elusive and controversial. Briefly, I will discuss some of these studies and their implications for more abstract notions such as the self and its place in the study of the brain. Additionally, I will provide some recent data demonstrating that EEG LORETA can be used to evaluate the cortical mechanisms (or networks) involved in psychological assessment procedures. In my view, this is one of the more important areas for study, such that if we continue to add to the armamentarium of psychological evaluation instruments it is imperative that we begin to invest in the neural morphology of these constructs.

The neural morphology of working memory and processing speed as measured by intelligence tests has yet to be investigated. However, we have numerous studies investigating these processes in prior chapters. I will provide brief examples from a set of data from our studies of LORETA neurofeedback in the AC and bilateral PFC. The primary assumption associated with this data is that LNFB was the differentiating factor in the increase in both cognitive domains between pre and post training. With this in mind we took the obtained scores from the WAIS-III processing speed index scores (PSI) and working memory index scores (WMI) and ran correlation analyses to determine the associations between the seven regions of interest, frequency domain current source density and the obtained scores as a result of LNFB in three different regions of training (AC, LPFC, RPFC). Figure 59 shows the results for the correlation analyses between WMI and PSI by region and frequency by each region of training.

The regions of interest from Figure 48 in chapter 4 are depicted within the graphs. The associated network features shown in Figures 53, 54, and 56 are also important for interpreting these results. In the graph, only coefficient values > .200 are considered significant <.01, additionally the sample size for the groups are different and further research is needed; however, these are very interesting results nonetheless. The correlations between the obtained scores in the AC group indicate differential and potential preferential relationships. The trained frequency (low-beta) and delta nearly appear to share a positive association with the scores except for arithmetic.

Theta, alpha-1, and alpha-2, on the other hand, show more negative associations with scores in many of the regions with the exceptions of arithmetic, symbol search, and digit-span. The beta frequency however, shows positive associations between scores in nearly all regions. The LPFC group shows some similarity with the AC group; however, noticeable differences are apparent. The trained frequency shows negative correlations for coding, arithmetic and letter number subtests. In delta, only positive associations are shown between LPFC, letter number and symbol search. Alpha-1 and alpha-2 show significant positive associations with letter number and coding in nearly all of the regions. Beta on the other hand shows significant positive associations with all subtests with the exception of coding.

The RPFC group shows the most dramatic associations, both positive and negative, between the variables. The trained frequency, delta, theta and beta show positive associations between region, frequency and subtest scores, with negative associations in beta for coding. Alpha-1 and alpha-2 show a dramatic negative association with all subtest scores in all regions of interest. It may be that this specific effect in the RPFC is associated with the saliency of the stimuli and attentional regulation via the relationship between the RFPC, RPCG, LPFC, and AC, with the AC performing some specific gating effect between the cortex, thalamic, limbic and brain-stem mechanisms.

Figure 60 (next 3 pages): Correlations between WMI and PSI scores by region and frequency. From top to bottom are the frequency domains top = TF (14 - 18 Hz), Delta (0.5 - 3.5 Hz), Theta (3.5 - 8.0 Hz), Alpha-1 (8.0 - 10.0 Hz), Alpha-2 (10.0 - 12.0 Hz) and beta (12.0 - 32.0 Hz). From left to right the columns are arranged by region of training AC, LPFC and RPFC. Within the graphs, the bars represent the subtests of the WMI and PSI. The WMI consists of the arithmetic, digit-span and letter-number sequencing subtests. The PSI consists of the symbol search and coding subtests. On the abscissa are the seven regions of interest we analyzed in our study. These were apriori ROIs and as such, we only examine the correlations between these regions and the subtest scores with the assumption that more widespread network functions are involved. On the ordinate is the Pearson correlation coefficient for the analyses. In short the graph illustrates potential frequency*region*cognitive function patterns that may have been directly influenced by LNFB in a specific region of training. This is a focus for our current research projects with ADHD and the precuneus.

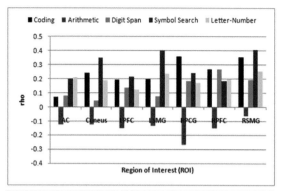

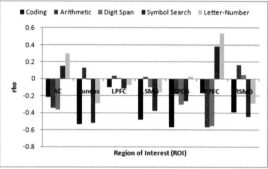

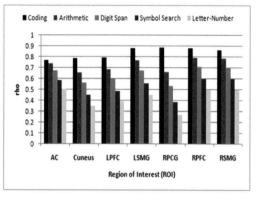

TF = (14-18 Hz)

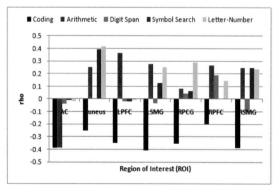

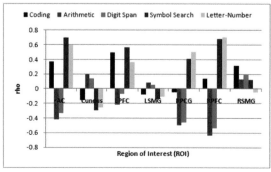

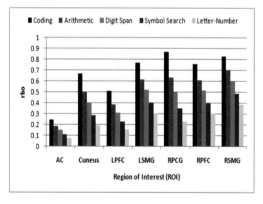

Delta = (0.5-3.5 Hz)

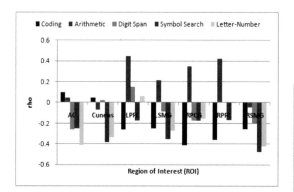

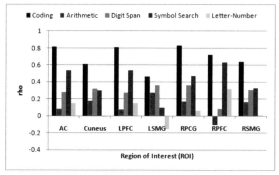

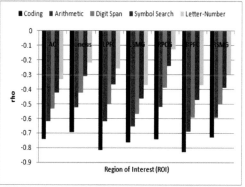

Theta = (3.5-8.0 Hz)

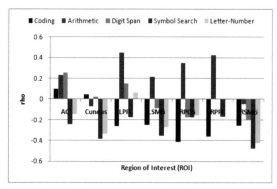

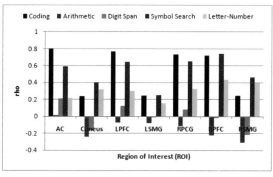

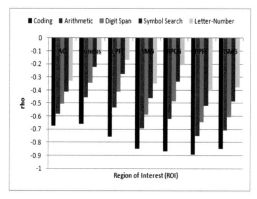

Alpha-1 = (8.0-10.0 Hz)

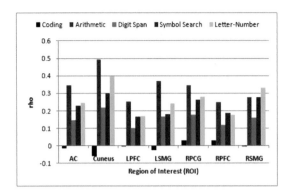

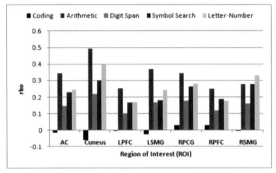

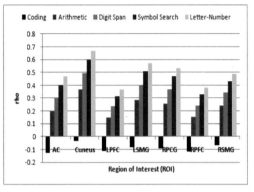

Alpha-2 = (10.0-12.0 Hz)

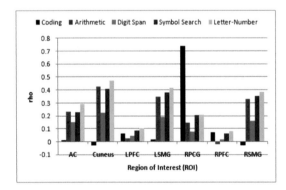

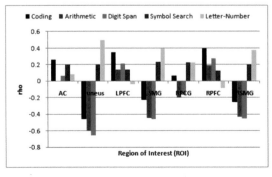

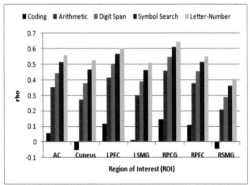

Beta = (12.0-32.0 Hz)

Spatial-specific cortical mapping and operant conditioning of the EEG current source density is quickly emerging as an important area of investigation (Cannon et al., 2007, 2009). Functional mapping of the relationships between cortical regions will eventually provide important insight into the morphology of numerous cognitive and affective processes, in addition to dysfunctional syndromes (Zanto, Toy, & Gazzaley, 2010; Rypma et al., 2006; Waiter et al., 2009). The use of intelligence indices and subtests, such as digit-symbol substitution and verbal fluency, to measure processing efficiency and working memory are well established (Brebion et al., 2000; Rypma et al., 2006; Salthouse, 1996; Turken et al., 2008). These types of studies have been conducted in various populations, such as brain-injury, normal aging, and Alzheimer's disease (AD) (Dos Santos et al., 2011; Mattay et al., 2006; Turken et al., 2008). Morphological studies conducted on populations suffering from neurodegenerative diseases provide a strong basis for hypotheses on functional cortical correlates. For instance, both MRI and manual segmentation studies have found an association between reduced verbal fluency and reduced gray matter in the left prefrontal cortices (Dos Santos et al., 2011; Fama et al., 1997; Pantel et al., 2004).

In recent years, the study of functional connectivity within the brain consists of complex measurements using a variety of techniques, including correlation analyses, partial correlation procedures, diffusion tensor imaging, and path analyses. It has become more than apparent that the localization myth cannot endure; instead, it can be modified such that specific regions within the brain may perform a specific function; however, it is unlikely that they perform these functions in a singular manner. Rather, it performs this function within and between networks. Patterns of cortical lateralization can vary along both the magnitude and the direction of hemispheric specialization (Galaburda, 1995). The magnitude of lateralization is often discussed in terms of interhemispheric connectivity and communication, while the direction of lateralization is conceptualized in terms of intrahemispheric organization (Zaidel et al., 1995). While decades of research with normal and clinical human populations has led to theories that postulate a left hemisphere specialization for language: communicative functioning and a right hemisphere specialization for processing spatial information, individual differences in patterns of cerebral lateralization are noted in terms of both the direction and degree of specialization (Hellige, 1990).

Nearly all neurocognitive behaviors depend on the cooperative and integrative functioning of the left and right cerebral hemispheres (Hellige, 1993). The left hemisphere (LH) and right hemisphere (RH) are thought to differ at the level of data-dependent computational-integration used to process information of all types, such that very few, if any neurocognitive functions are performed singularly by region or hemisphere. It is however, evident that when a task favors the computational bias of one hemisphere, performance or state-dependent asymmetries are likely to result.

These asymmetries are evidenced by the differential effects of left and right unilateral brain injury and by differing performance profiles for stimuli presented to the left or right hemispheres in neurologically normal or split-brain individuals (Hellige, 1993; Zaidel, 1978). Cummings proposed (Cummings, 1997) three approaches to evaluating the neuropsychiatry of right brain dysfunction: (1) assessment of conditions that follow the occurrence of right brain damage and have the symptoms of traditional psychiatric conditions such as depression, mania, psychosis, hallucinations, anxiety, and dissociation; (2) investigation of syndromes that are not easily classified as conventional psychiatric disorders but occur with right brain injuries and impact personal behavior and interpersonal interactions (including disorders of facial and vocal recognition, abnormalities of emotional vocal and facial expression, and the neglect and anosognosia syndromes); and (3) evaluation of right brain function in patients with conventional psychiatric diagnoses and no evidence of acquired brain injury (depression, bipolar illness, schizophrenia, anxiety, etc.).

Disorders of the right hemisphere have been studied intensively for the past three decades and substantial advances have been made in understanding the neuropsychological functions of this cerebral region. Aspects of visuospatial function, visuomotor activity, visual discrimination and recognition, nonverbal memory, music, and prosody have been shown to be mediated by specialized functional regions within the right brain (Cummings, 1997). Thus one possible hypotheses for the data presented in Figure 59 is that each frequency domain may play an important role in the processing of information and the associated functions. For example, working memory and attention are interdependent processes, such that one function cannot exist in unimpaired fashion without the other.

In considering the graphs, it is evident that each of the seven regions plays a role in both working memory and processing speed tasks, as measured by the WMI and PSI of the WAIS-III. Increased neural involvement, paired with similar task accuracy between clinical and control groups, has been interpreted as "neural compensation" or, alternatively, as "brain reorganization". While these two terms certainly have distinct implications for altered brain activation, (most notably its permanence), both are almost universally used to describe PFC involvement operating to bolster performance (Hillary, 2008).

Contrarily, the data presented suggest that no one (e.g., PFC, DLPFC) region alone accounts for a specific cognitive function, rather numerous regions (networks) play a role in the process. Therefore, brain reorganization and neural plasticity may not be an isolated phenomenon (e.g. one region subsuming the function of another) – rather apriori experience dependent associations may exist in order to facilitate such a process.

Certainly, more advanced methods of analyses would be prudent in understanding these types of data and the relationship between these regions and frequencies with specific cognitive and affective tasks.

Figures 61 (below) and 62 (next page) show another example of cross-frequency coupling or the interdependency between EEG frequency domains in a single region of interest, in this case a seven voxel cluster or neurons in the AC. In the figures, from left to right and top to bottom, are the current source density levels for each frequency for ADHD, SUD, and eight normal controls resulting from LNFB in that region. The figures illustrate the Pearson rho on the y-axis, the frequency domains on the x-axis, and the frequency domains. The partial correlation analyses show the relationship between two frequencies, ruling out the effects of all other frequencies.

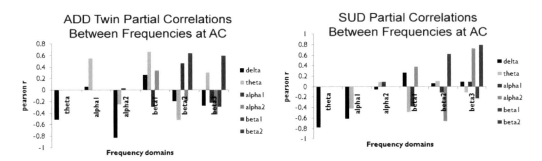

FREQUENCY SPECIFIC DISORDERS?

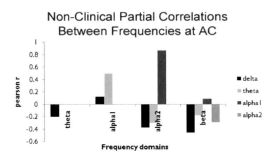

Figure 61: Partial correlations within the cluster of voxels for LNFB in three different populations. Within the charts on the x-axis are the frequency domains and the Pearson correlation coefficient for the partial procedure is on the y-axis. The top left shows the relationship between the EEG current source densities in the AC because of LNFB training. Clearly, there are positive and negative effects between the frequencies in this ROI in the ADHD twins. Theta shows a negative relationship with delta, alpha-1 shows a positive relationship with theta, alpha-2 shows a negative relationship with delta and theta, beta-1 shows a positive relationship with theta, delta and alpha-2, beta-2 shows a positive relationship with alpha-1 and beta-1 and a negative relationship with delta, theta and alpha-2. Beta-3 shows a positive relationship with beta- and theta and a negative relationship with delta, alpha-1, alpha-2 and beta-1. A recovering substance abuser using the same analysis in the AC is shown on the right. The relationship between the frequencies within the AC appears to have a specific pattern such that alpha-2 and delta show a positive relationship and a negative relationship with theta and alpha-1. Beta 1 shows a negative relationship with alpha-1 and theta while beta 2 shows a negative relationship with alpha-2. The lower graph is the normal population. Theta shows a positive relationship with apha-1, alpha-1 shows a positive relationship with beta shows a negative relationship with delta, theta and alpha-2.

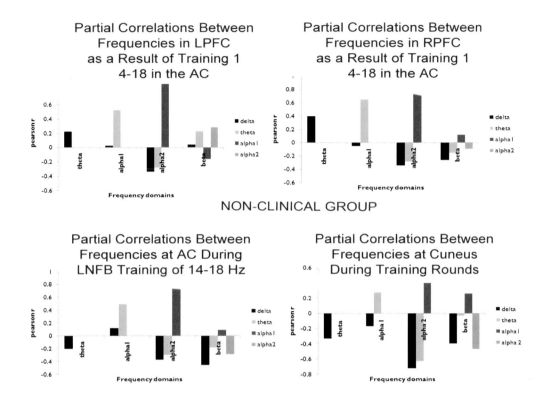

Figure 62: Partial correlations between the EEG CSD within four regions of interest in our LNFB study. In the figure from left to right and top to bottom are the regions of interest LPFC, RPFC, AC and Cuneus. Within the graphs are the frequency domains - delta, theta, alpha-1, alpha-2 and beta. On the y-axis is the Pearson correlation coefficient for the partial procedure. There are clear similarities between anterior regions, with subtle but significant differences between the 3 frontal ROI. The cuneus on the other hand is much different from anterior regions but still maintains similarities that could possibly represent a method of signal communication and modulation between these regions. Further research into this method is certainly of interest and mathematical models and computational methods are under development in our lab as well as others.

Experience-dependent changes in the human brain can occur from a synaptic to a cortical level throughout the life span (Holloway, 2003). There is a growing literature base demonstrating these neuroplasticity effects in both human and non-human populations. I tend to think of neuroplasticity in terms of development, such that in our earliest periods of development we assimilate information because of learning (operant behavior) by mimicking, observing, and experiencing the environment. We also begin to organize the self critically based on our perceptions of self in relation to others (operant behavior driven by self-perception and its relation to the environment). As development progresses, so does the data-dependency requirements on the brain through which we learn to adapt in an operantly efficient way (the result of learning, practice and specialization). In essence, development is a function of operant learning, and disorders of learning begin and end with the central nervous system and its functional integrity. In adulthood, we continually update and add to the data-dependency, which increases the operant efficiency. This may also be thought of in terms of executive functions and self-regulation. These two definitions are synonymous and described with functional neural signatures (e.g., functional integrity of the CNS). It is when some data dependency module (negative self-perception, abuse, affect regulation or deficits in self-regulation) relative to the self occurs that problems in operant efficiency and psychological well-being are compromised. It is reasonable to consider that the self (organized neural networks) is both malleable and in some aspects more resistant to the effects of new learning (i.e., religion, disciplines, values, morality). Executive functions and self-regulation are the predominant focus of treatment for many disorders (e.g., depression, anxiety, SUD).

It may also be that there are specific genetic mechanisms associated with the homeostatic module of the organism that become disorganized or skewed toward a negative data-selection process. I tend to conceptualize it within this framework Behavioral Equilibrium (or Operant Efficiency) is dependent (on the output) on the interaction between emotional equilibrium (EE) and homeostasis (HS) or BE = EE/HS. The mediating variable for Operant Efficiency or Operant Inefficiency is self-regulation (SR) or its equivalent executive functions (EF). The primary assumption underlying this model is neuroplasticity. Neuroplasticity is the inherent capacity of the brain to develop new connections as a compensatory mechanism for injury or as a function of learning in response to experience and changes in the environment. Clearly, neuroplasticity is the driving force in human learning (experience dependent changes) over the lifespan. This experience-driven effect has refuted the long help position that the adult human brain is both hardwired and resistant to change (Holloway, 2003). Experience-driven changes have been widely demonstrated in both human and non-human primates and these findings present exceptional challenges to find specific tasks elucidating how these mechanisms occur and to develop methods to influence these processes to aid in the development of effective treatments for disorders of learning (OE). For example, a large body of literature has demonstrated that compromised functional integrity of networks within the brains of individuals with ADHD, SUD, MDD, AD, ASD, and nearly every other psychiatric/psychological disorder (Barry et al., 2010; Barry, Clarke, McCarthy, & Selikowitz, 2002; Berman et al., 2010; Bluhm et al., 2009; Bluhm et al., 2008; Cannon, 2009; Fair et al., 2010a, 2010b; Grady et al., 2009; Gusnard et al., 2001; Hale et al., 2010; Hung et al., 2010; Just, Cherkassky, Keller, Kana, & Minshew, 2007; Navarro et al., 2002; Peterson et al., 2009; Pizzagalli et al., 2001; Sambataro et al., 2008; Santesso et al., 2008; Seminowicz et al., 2004; Sheline et al., 2009; Sperling et al., 2009; Stevens, Pearlson, & Kiehl, 2007; Sumich et al., 2009; Tamm, Menon, & Reiss, 2006; Thibodeau et al., 2006; Tian et al., 2006; Yerys et al., 2009).

There is little doubt that symptoms associated with these disorders can be attributed to functional network disruptions, regional activation patterns and lack of the functional integration of systems required for OE. Practicing cognitive tasks is proposed to increase the efficiency of the distributed network associated with the specific task that typically is reflected by a decrease in activity in the network of neural assemblies underlying task performance. Studies examining the effects of cognitive tasks associated with working memory, visuo-spatial, verbal fluency, and object-spatial processing have shown consistent decreased activity associated with practice and learning, as have numerous studies investigating musical practice and motor skills. This pattern is consistent with neurophysiological research in non-human primates that showed weaker neuronal activity in response to practiced or familiar stimuli or task conditions.

Decreases in the extent or intensity of activations are observed in the majority of studies examining task practice. The primary mechanism proposed to underlie activation decreases is increased neural efficiency, which by definition reflects an increased efficiency within a network such that operant efficiency now occurs with the engagement of fewer neural sources and increased synchronous firing relative to a particular task or stimulus (Foerde et al., 2008; Poldrack, 2002; Poldrack, Desmond, Glover, & Gabrieli, 1998; Poldrack & Gabrieli, 2001; Poldrack, Selco, Field, & Cohen, 1999). Decreases in activation is suggested to represent a more robust and efficient neural representation (Duncan & Miller, 2002) or a more precise functional circuit (Garavan et al., 2000). In several studies of practice effects in the brain, increases in activation refer to two processes practice-related expansions in the volume of cortical representations and increases in the strength or amplitude of activations. The role of neuroplasticity in this theory is based on cognitive tasks that show specific activations or deactivations as an effect of practice and learning, treatment effects of cognitive behavioral therapy and other treatment models that have shown pre-post changes in the cortical landscape. Similar changes in this landscape have been shown in studies of neurofeedback. The fundamental process underlying all neuromodulation techniques, regardless of method is neuroplasticity.

It may be advantageous to utilize gain and spectral analysis as measures of learning between cortical units. The gain value is computed by dividing the cross-amplitude value by the spectrum density estimates for one of the two series in the analysis. Consequently, two gain values are computed, which can be interpreted as the standard least squares regression coefficients for the respective frequencies. Numerous analytic components are involved in time series applications.

For ease of communicating the effects of LNFB and learning, I will focus on the gain measure between two regions for control subjects and an ADHD subject with an equal number of sessions. We wanted to know how the two regions interact across time during the training rounds in order to understand better the mechanisms through which operant conditioning of self-regulation manifests. Figure 63 (pgs 201-202) shows the gain for the mean 14 - 18 Hz for the normal subjects (left) and an ADHD subject (right) for 30 sessions of LNFB in the AC. From top to bottom in the figure are the gain measures between AC*LPFC, AC*RPFC, LPFC*RPFC and AC*Cuneus. On the x-axis are the sessions 1, 5, 10, 15, 20, and 25 and on the y-axis is the gain value (SLS regression coefficients for the sessions).

In essence, the graphs demonstrate the learning effect of LNFB between the AC and each of the regions. Intuitively, we would expect a significant relationship between the AC and regions within a network to be influenced by LNFB training, which can be thought of as both practice and operant learning associated with the neural sources of self-regulation and attention. As such, and with the sample size considered, there is clear evidence of learning between the regions in the normal subjects; however, the ADHD individual, despite the learning curve shown in the earlier chapter does not produce the integrative effect or network training as is shown in the normative sample comparisons. These effects in the AC and LPFC have consistently been shown in studies of prefrontal and default network studies with additional evidence of a parietal disconnection in ADHD.

The effects of gain and phase during classical conditioning experiments have been shown between neurons in the orbital frontal cortex and amygdala as well as single cell studies showing classical conditioning effects in the lateral amygdala in the rat (Clugnet & LeDoux, 1990; Clugnet, LeDoux, & Morrison, 1990; LeDoux, Cicchetti, Xagoraris, & Romanski, 1990; LeDoux, Farb, & Ruggiero, 1990). Further research has demonstrated the role of the AC in conflict, competition and reward anticipation while other regions, namely the left parahippocampal gyrus, ventral striatum and left inferior frontal gyrus, showed the largest effect for reward magnitude (Alexander & Brown, 2010).

Neurons in the monkey striatum have been shown to respond to reward expectation and motor behaviors associated with the reward delivery (Apicella, Scarnati, Ljungberg, & Schultz, 1992; Ljungberg, Apicella, & Schultz, 1992). Studies of the human striatum have reported increased activity during both primary and secondary reward processing (Kirsch et al., 2003; Pagnoni, Zink, Montague, & Berns, 2002). Striatal responses to the anticipation and delivery of rewards and punishments implicate it in the operant behavior model described earlier in the text such that inputs from affective, cognitive and motor networks would be involved in reward and the associated reinforcement (stimulus-event). Interestingly, the caudate, as part of the dorsal striatum responds more preferentially to the action associated with reinforcement and reward especially in circumstances where predictions and feedback are used to modify behavior (Tricomi, Delgado, & Fiez, 2004). It is proposed that the plastic properties of the striatum permits a rapid reinforcement of actions as shown in synaptic changes during the learning of a procedural task (Jog, Kubota, Connolly, Hillegaart, & Graybiel, 1999) as well as tasks involving self-stimulation (Wickens, Reynolds, & Hyland, 2003). The caudate may play an important role in reinforcement and monitoring actions that produce reward as well as the ability to learn through reinforcement, which is the fundamental backdrop of operant conditioning (Delgado, Miller, Inati, & Phelps, 2005). Interestingly, the caudate has also been reported as increased in activity in studies of EEG biofeedback (neurofeedback) in children with ADHD (Beauregard & Levesque, 2006; Levesque, Beauregard, & Mensour, 2006). The ventral striatum is also implicated in emotion and motivational processes (Cardinal, Parkinson, Hall, & Everitt, 2002).

Given the large data demonstrating plasticity in the human brain, the question arises as to the long term potentiation and how neural pathways change or remain resistant to change based on negative self-reinforcement, negative self-perception, and negative self-world view (e.g., negative self-talk, negative self-view, low self-worth, etc.). This is certainly an area of interest in numerous psychiatric syndromes.

Controls 14-18 Hz CSD Across Sessions

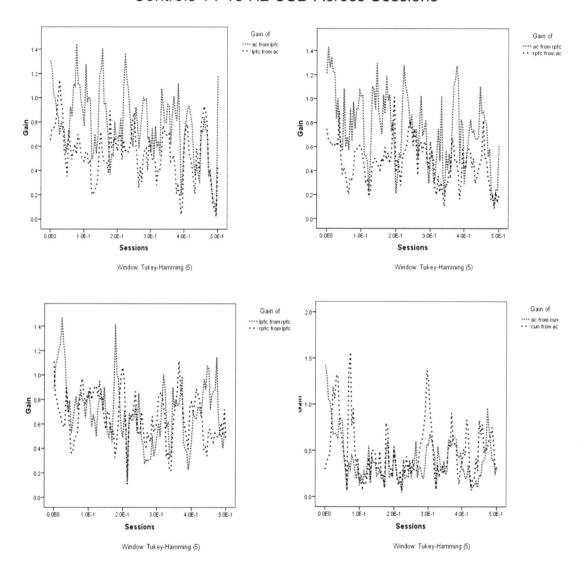

Figure 63 (above and next page): Spectral gain for the mean of 14 - 18 Hz for the normal subjects (left) and an ADHD subject (right) for 30 sessions of LNFB in the AC. From top to bottom in the figure are the gain measures between AC*LPFC, AC*RPFC, LPFC*RPFC and AC*Cuneus. On the x-axis are the sessions 1, 5, 10, 15, 20, 25 and on the y-axis is the gain value (SLS regression coefficients across sessions) for the sessions (or frequency).

ADHD 14-18 Hz Across Sessions

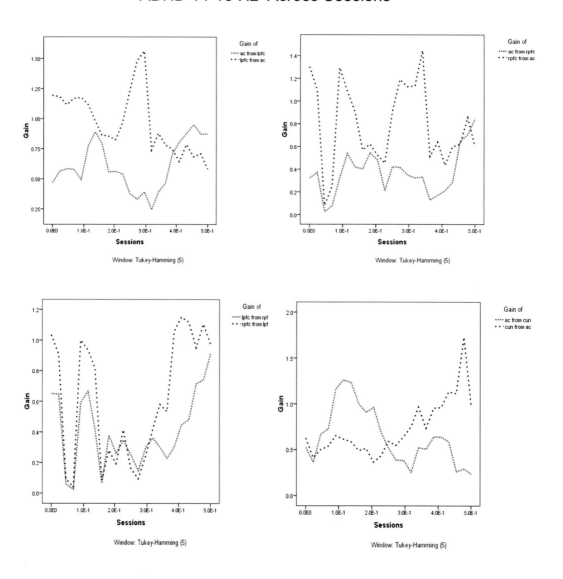

LORETA and EEG provide a means to examine the electrical activity of the brain and its sources in detail, and as such can only provide a benefit to other neuroimaging techniques. As technology progresses, so will the questions to be answered by neuroscience. Neuroplasticity and learning are but one example of processes that present significant challenges across disciplines. However, we can be reassured that the current methods will refute many prior notions and provide new theoretical and scientific methods to improve our research methods and clinical techniques.

7.1: Summary

LORETA and EEG provide a means to examine the electrical activity of the brain and its sources in detail, and as such can only provide a benefit to other neuroimaging techniques. As technology progresses, so will the questions to be answered by neuroscience. Neuroplasticity and learning are but one example of processes that present significant challenges across disciplines. However, we can be reassured that the current methods will refute many prior notions and provide new theoretical and scientific methods to improve our research methods and clinical techniques. Much of the data and interpretations presented in this chapter are novel and require extensive thought and rigorous interpretation. I am hard pressed to maintain an objective stance and voice when discussing novel approaches. Additionally, I strive to locate references for the findings I encounter to support the conclusions given. One of the most profound issues I struggle with is the neglect by many disciplines of science of experience-dependent (or data-dependent) plasticity. To sum this notion up, I can say without exception, the only reason I have written this book or do the research that I do is because I have sufficient data to do so. Every human being operates within his or her respective data, which is a direct function of learning (operant behavior or operating effectively on the environment). It is this data dependency that accounts for individual differences, unless a defect in the central nervous system exists. Understanding the organization of this data and the mechanisms of its processing is a topic of extreme interest to me. Again, I say these are exciting times for all disciplines devoted to understanding this organ we call brain.

BIBLIOGRAPHY

Abrahams, S., Goldstein, L. H., Simmons, A., Brammer, M. J., Williams, S. C., Giampietro, V. P., et al. (2003). Functional magnetic resonance imaging of verbal fluency and confrontation naming using compressed image acquisition to permit overt responses. *Hum Brain Mapp, 20*(1), 29-40.

Adinoff, B. (2004). Neurobiologic processes in drug reward and addiction. *Harv Rev Psychiatry, 12*(6), 305-320.

Aguirre-Perez, D. M., Otero-Ojeda, G. A., Pliego-Rivero, F. B., & Ferreira-Martinez, A. A. (2007). Relationship of working memory and EEG to academic performance: a study among high school students. *Int J Neurosci, 117*(6), 869-882.

Akila, R., Muller, K., Kaukiainen, A., & Sainio, M. (2006). Memory performance profile in occupational chronic solvent encephalopathy suggests working memory dysfunction. *J Clin Exp Neuropsychol, 28*(8), 1307-1326.

Alexander, M., & Rosen, R. C. (2008). Spinal cord injuries and orgasm: a review. J *Sex Marital Ther, 34*(4), 308-324.

Alexander, W. H., & Brown, J. W. (2010). Competition between learned reward and error outcome predictions in anterior cingulate cortex. *Neuroimage, 49*(4), 3210-3218.

Allman, J. M., Hakeem, A., Erwin, J. M., Nimchinsky, E., & Hof, P. (2001). The anterior cingulate cortex. The evolution of an interface between emotion and cognition. *Ann N Y Acad Sci, 935*, 107-117.

Alonso-Deflorida, F., & Delgado, J. M. (1958). Lasting behavioral and EEG changes in cats induced by prolonged stimulation of amygdala. *Am J Physiol, 193*(1), 223-229.

Alper, K. R. (1999). The EEG and cocaine sensitization: a hypothesis. *J Neuropsychiatry Clin Neurosci, 11*(2), 209-221.

Alper, K. R., Chabot, R. J., Kim, A. H., Prichep, L. S., & John, E. R. (1990). Quantitative EEG correlates of crack cocaine dependence. *Psychiatry Res, 35*(2), 95-105.

Amunts, K., Weiss, P. H., Mohlberg, H., Pieperhoff, P., Eickhoff, S., Gurd, J. M., et al. (2004). Analysis of neural mechanisms underlying verbal fluency in cytoarchitectonically defined stereotaxic space--the roles of Brodmann areas 44 and 45. *Neuroimage, 22*(1), 42-56.

Anderer, P., Saletu, B., Semlitsch, H. V., & Pascual-Marqui, R. D. (2003). Non-invasive localization of P300 sources in normal aging and age-associated memory impairment. *Neurobiol Aging, 24*(3), 463-479.

Angelakis, E., Lubar, J. F., & Stathopoulou, S. (2004). Electroencephalographic peak alpha frequency correlates of cognitive traits. *Neurosci Lett, 371*(1), 60-63.

Angelakis, E., Lubar, J. F., Stathopoulou, S., & Kounios, J. (2004). Peak alpha frequency: an electroencephalographic measure of cognitive preparedness. *Clin Neurophysiol, 115*(4), 887-897.

Angelakis, E., Stathopoulou, S., Frymiare, J. L., Green, D. L., Lubar, J. F., & Kounios, J. (2007). EEG neurofeedback: a brief overview and an example of peak alpha frequency training for cognitive enhancement in the elderly. *Clin Neuropsychol, 21*(1), 110-129.

Apicella, P., Scarnati, E., Ljungberg, T., & Schultz, W. (1992). Neuronal activity in monkey striatum related to the expectation of predictable environmental events. *J Neurophysiol, 68*(3), 945-960.

Araujo, L., Goldberg, P., Eyma, J., Madhusoodanan, S., Buff, D. D., Shamim, K., et al. (1996). The effect of anxiety and depression on completion/withdrawal status in patients admitted to substance abuse detoxification program. *J Subst Abuse Treat, 13*(1), 61-66.

Arnone, D., Barrick, T. R., Chengappa, S., Mackay, C. E., Clark, C. A., & Abou-Saleh, M. T. (2008). Corpus callosum damage in heavy marijuana use: preliminary evidence from diffusion tensor tractography and tract-based spatial statistics. *Neuroimage, 41*(3), 1067-1074.

Arns, M., de Ridder, S., Strehl, U., Breteler, M., & Coenen, A. (2009). Efficacy of neurofeedback treatment in ADHD: the effects on inattention, impulsivity and hyperactivity: a meta-analysis. *Clin EEG Neurosci, 40*(3), 180-189.

Arnsten, A. F. (2006). Stimulants: Therapeutic actions in ADHD. *Neuropsychopharmacology, 31*(11), 2376-2383.

Averill, J. R. (1983). Studies on anger and aggression. Implications for theories of emotion. *Am Psychol, 38*(11), 1145-1160.

Awad, M., Warren, J. E., Scott, S. K., Turkheimer, F. E., & Wise, R. J. (2007). A common system for the comprehension and production of narrative speech. *J Neurosci, 27*(43), 11455-11464.

Babiloni, C., Babiloni, F., Carducci, F., Cincotti, F., Vecchio, F., Cola, B., et al. (2004). Functional frontoparietal connectivity during short-term memory as revealed by high-resolution EEG coherence analysis. *Behav Neurosci, 118*(4), 687-697.

Babiloni, C., Frisoni, G., Steriade, M., Bresciani, L., Binetti, G., Del Percio, C., et al. (2006). Frontal white matter volume and delta EEG sources negatively correlate in awake subjects with mild cognitive impairment and Alzheimer's disease. Clin Neurophysiol, 117(5), 1113-1129.

Ballmaier, M., Toga, A. W., Blanton, R. E., Sowell, E. R., Lavretsky, H., Peterson, J., et al. (2004). Anterior cingulate, gyrus rectus, and orbitofrontal abnormalities in elderly depressed patients: an MRI-based parcellation of the prefrontal cortex. Am J Psychiatry, 161(1), 99-108.

Barch, D. M. (2005). The cognitive neuroscience of schizophrenia. Annu Rev Clin Psychol, 1, 321-353.

Barde, L. H., & Thompson-Schill, S. L. (2002). Models of functional organization of the lateral prefrontal cortex in verbal working memory: evidence in favor of the process model. J Cogn Neurosci, 14(7), 1054-1063.

Barry, R. J., Clarke, A. R., Hajos, M., McCarthy, R., Selikowitz, M., & Dupuy, F. E. (2010). Resting-state EEG gamma activity in children with attention-deficit/hyperactivity disorder. Clin Neurophysiol, 121(11), 1871-1877.

Barry, R. J., Clarke, A. R., McCarthy, R., & Selikowitz, M. (2002). EEG coherence in attention-deficit/hyperactivity disorder: a comparative study of two DSM-IV types. Clin Neurophysiol, 113(4), 579-585.

Basar, E., Basar-Eroglu, C., Karakas, S., & Schurmann, M. (1999). Oscillatory brain theory: a new trend in neuroscience. IEEE Eng Med Biol Mag, 18(3), 56-66.

Basar, E., Basar-Eroglu, C., Karakas, S., & Schurmann, M. (2001). Gamma, alpha, delta, and theta oscillations govern cognitive processes. Int J Psychophysiol, 39(2-3), 241-248.

Bast, T. (2007). Toward an integrative perspective on hippocampal function: from the rapid encoding of experience to adaptive behavior. Rev Neurosci, 18(3-4), 253-281.

Bastiaansen, M. C., van der Linden, M., Ter Keurs, M., Dijkstra, T., & Hagoort, P. (2005). Theta responses are involved in lexical-semantic retrieval during language processing. J Cogn Neurosci, 17(3), 530-541.

Batson, H. W., Brown, L. S., Jr., Zaballero, A. R., Chu, A., & Alterman, A. I. (1993). Conflicting measurements of depression in a substance abuse population. J Subst Abuse, 5(1), 93-100.

Bauer, L. O. (2001). Predicting relapse to alcohol and drug abuse via quantitative electroencephalography. Neuropsychopharmacology, 25(3), 332-340.

Bauer, T. M., Steinbruckner, B., Brinkmann, F. E., Ditzen, A. K., Schwacha, H., Aponte, J. J., et al. (2001). Small intestinal bacterial overgrowth in patients with cirrhosis: prevalence and relation with spontaneous bacterial peritonitis. Am J Gastroenterol, 96(10), 2962-2967.

Baxter, L. R., Jr., Schwartz, J. M., Bergman, K. S., Szuba, M. P., Guze, B. H., Mazziotta, J. C., et al. (1992). Caudate glucose metabolic rate changes with both drug and behavior therapy for obsessive-compulsive disorder. Arch Gen Psychiatry, 49(9), 681-689.

Beasley, C. L., Pennington, K., Behan, A., Wait, R., Dunn, M. J., & Cotter, D. (2006). Proteomic analysis of the anterior cingulate cortex in the major psychiatric disorders: Evidence for disease-associated changes. *Proteomics*, 6(11), 3414-3425.

Beauregard, M., & Levesque, J. (2006). Functional magnetic resonance imaging investigation of the effects of neurofeedback training on the neural bases of selective attention and response inhibition in children with attention-deficit/hyperactivity disorder. *Appl Psychophysiol Biofeedback*, 31(1), 3-20.

Beauregard, M., Levesque, J., & Bourgouin, P. (2001). Neural correlates of conscious self-regulation of emotion. *J Neurosci*, 21(18), RC165.

Beck, A. T. (1964). Thinking and Depression. Ii. Theory and Therapy. *Arch Gen Psychiatry*, 10, 561-571.

Beck, A. T. (2008). The evolution of the cognitive model of depression and its neurobiological correlates. *Am J Psychiatry*, 165(8), 969-977.

Beck, A. T., Hollon, S. D., Young, J. E., Bedrosian, R. C., & Budenz, D. (1985). Treatment of depression with cognitive therapy and amitriptyline. *Arch Gen Psychiatry*, 42(2), 142-148.

Beck, A. T., & Rush, A. J. (1985). A cognitive model of anxiety formation and anxiety resolution. *Issues Ment Health Nurs*, 7(1-4), 349-365.

Beckmann, H., & Jakob, H. (1991). Prenatal disturbances of nerve cell migration in the entorhinal region: a common vulnerability factor in functional psychoses? *J Neural Transm Gen Sect*, 84(1-2), 155-164.

Bench, C. J., Friston, K. J., Brown, R. G., Scott, L. C., Frackowiak, R. S., & Dolan, R. J. (1992). The anatomy of melancholia--focal abnormalities of cerebral blood flow in major depression. *Psychol Med*, 22(3), 607-615.

Bench, C. J., Frith, C. D., Grasby, P. M., Friston, K. J., Paulesu, E., Frackowiak, R. S., et al. (1993). Investigations of the functional anatomy of attention using the Stroop test. *Neuropsychologia*, 31(9), 907-922.

Bendat, J. S., and Piersol, A.G (2001). *Random Data: Analysis and Measurement Procedures* (3rd ed.). New York: Wiley.

Berger, H. (1929). Über das Elektroenkephalogram des Menschen. *Arch. f. Psychiat.*, 87, 527 - 570.

Berman, M. G., Peltier, S., Nee, D. E., Kross, E., Deldin, P. J., & Jonides, J. (2010). Depression, rumination and the default network. *Soc Cogn Affect Neurosci.* 6:548-555

Berthoz, S., Armony, J. L., Blair, R. J., & Dolan, R. J. (2002). An fMRI study of intentional and unintentional (embarrassing) violations of social norms. *Brain*, 125(Pt 8), 1696-1708.

Biederman, J., Wilens, T., Mick, E., Milberger, S., Spencer, T. J., & Faraone, S. V. (1995). Psychoactive substance use disorders in adults with attention deficit hyperactivity disorder (ADHD): effects of ADHD and psychiatric comorbidity. *Am J Psychiatry*, 152(11), 1652-1658.

Bihrle, A. M., Brownell, H. H., Powelson, J. A., & Gardner, H. (1986). Comprehension of humorous and nonhumorous materials by left and right brain-damaged patients. *Brain Cogn*, 5(4), 399-411.

Birbaumer, N., Grodd, W., Diedrich, O., Klose, U., Erb, M., Lotze, M., et al. (1998). fMRI reveals amygdala activation to human faces in social phobics. *Neuroreport*, 9(6), 1223-1226.

Bjork, M. H., Sand, T., Brathen, G., Linaker, O. M., Morken, G., Nilsen, B. M., et al. (2008). Quantitative EEG findings in patients with acute, brief depression combined with other fluctuating psychiatric symptoms: a controlled study from an acute psychiatric department. *BMC Psychiatry*, 8, 89.

Blair, R. J. (2007). The amygdala and ventromedial prefrontal cortex in morality and psychopathy. *Trends Cogn Sci*, 11(9), 387-392.

Bleich, S., Bandelow, B., Javaheripour, K., Muller, A., Degner, D., Wilhelm, J., et al. (2003). Hyperhomocysteinemia as a new risk factor for brain shrinkage in patients with alcoholism. *Neurosci Lett*, 335(3), 179-182.

Bleich, S., Sperling, W., Degner, D., Graesel, E., Bleich, K., Wilhelm, J., et al. (2003). Lack of association between hippocampal volume reduction and first-onset alcohol withdrawal seizure. A volumetric MRI study. *Alcohol Alcohol*, 38(1), 40-44.

Bleich, S., Wilhelm, J., Graesel, E., Degner, D., Sperling, W., Rossner, V., et al. (2003). Apolipoprotein E epsilon 4 is associated with hippocampal volume reduction in females with alcoholism. *J Neural Transm*, 110(4), 401-411.

Bluhm, R., Williamson, P., Lanius, R., Theberge, J., Densmore, M., Bartha, R., et al. (2009). Resting state default-mode network connectivity in early depression using a seed region-of-interest analysis: decreased connectivity with caudate nucleus. *Psychiatry Clin Neurosci*, 63(6), 754-761.

Bluhm, R. L., Osuch, E. A., Lanius, R. A., Boksman, K., Neufeld, R. W., Theberge, J., et al. (2008). Default mode network connectivity: effects of age, sex, and analytic approach. *Neuroreport*, 19(8), 887-891.

Bolton, E., & Calhoun, C. L. (1971). The concept and misconception of homonymous hemianopsia. A case of the parietal lobe syndrome. *J Natl Med Assoc*, 63(6), 441-444.

Borst, J. G., Leung, L. W., & MacFabe, D. F. (1987). Electrical activity of the cingulate cortex. II. Cholinergic modulation. *Brain Res*, 407(1), 81-93.

Bouma, E. M., Riese, H., Ormel, J., Verhulst, F. C., & Oldehinkel, A. J. (2009). Adolescents' cortisol responses to awakening and social stress; Effects of gender, menstrual phase and oral contraceptives. The TRAILS study. *Psychoneuroendocrinology*, 34(6), 884-893.

Boutros, N. N., Mears, R., Pflieger, M. E., Moxon, K. A., Ludowig, E., & Rosburg, T. (2007). Sensory gating in the human hippocampal and rhinal regions: Regional differences. *Hippocampus.*18:310-316

Braak, H., & Braak, E. (1985). On areas of transition between entorhinal allocortex and temporal isocortex in the human brain. Normal morphology and lamina-specific pathology in Alzheimer's disease. *Acta Neuropathol*, 68(4), 325-332.

Brady, N., Campbell, M., & Flaherty, M. (2004). My left brain and me: a dissociation in the perception of self and others. *Neuropsychologia*, 42(9), 1156-1161.

Brazdil, M., Babiloni, C., Roman, R., Daniel, P., Bares, M., Rektor, I., et al. (2007). Directional functional coupling of cerebral rhythms between anterior cingulate and dorsolateral prefrontal areas during rare stimuli: A directed transfer function analysis of human depth EEG signal. *Hum Brain Mapp.*30:138-146

Brazier, M. A. (1961). *A History of the Electrical Activity of the Brain*. The first half century. London: Pitman Medical Publishing Co.

Brazier, M. A. (1968). Studies of the EEG activity of limbic structures in man. *Electroencephalogr Clin Neurophysiol*, 25(4), 309-318.

Breiter, H. C., Rauch, S. L., Kwong, K. K., Baker, J. R., Weisskoff, R. M., Kennedy, D. N., et al. (1996). Functional magnetic resonance imaging of symptom provocation in obsessive-compulsive disorder. *Arch Gen Psychiatry*, 53(7), 595-606.

Bremner, J. D. (2007). Neuroimaging in Posttraumatic Stress Disorder and Other Stress-Related Disorders. *Neuroimaging Clin N Am*, 17(4), 523-538.

Breslau, N., Davis, G. C., Andreski, P., & Peterson, E. (1991). Traumatic events and posttraumatic stress disorder in an urban population of young adults. *Arch Gen Psychiatry*, 48(3), 216-222.

Brett, M., Johnsrude, I. S., & Owen, A. M. (2002). The problem of functional localization in the human brain. *Nat Rev Neurosci*, 3(3), 243-249.

Broderick, P. A. (1992). Cocaine's colocalized effects on synaptic serotonin and dopamine in ventral tegmentum in a reinforcement paradigm. *Pharmacol Biochem Behav*, 42(4), 889-898.

Brody, A. L., Saxena, S., Schwartz, J. M., Stoessel, P. W., Maidment, K., Phelps, M. E., et al. (1998). FDG-PET predictors of response to behavioral therapy and pharmacotherapy in obsessive compulsive disorder. *Psychiatry Res*, 84(1), 1-6.

Brown, P. J., Recupero, P. R., & Stout, R. (1995). PTSD substance abuse comorbidity and treatment utilization. *Addict Behav*, 20(2), 251-254.

Bruder, G. E., Fong, R., Tenke, C. E., Leite, P., Towey, J. P., Stewart, J. E., et al. (1997). Regional brain asymmetries in major depression with or without an anxiety disorder: a quantitative electroencephalographic study. *Biol Psychiatry,* 41(9), 939-948.

Bruder, G. E., Stewart, J. W., Mercier, M. A., Agosti, V., Leite, P., Donovan, S., et al. (1997). Outcome of cognitive-behavioral therapy for depression: relation to hemispheric dominance for verbal processing. *J Abnorm Psychol,* 106(1), 138-144.

Buchsbaum, M. S., Buchsbaum, B. R., Hazlett, E. A., Haznedar, M. M., Newmark, R., Tang, C. Y., et al. (2007). Relative glucose metabolic rate higher in white matter in patients with schizophrenia. *Am J Psychiatry,* 164(7), 1072-1081.

Buchsbaum, M. S., Haznedar, M., Newmark, R. E., Chu, K. W., Dusi, N., Entis, J. J., et al. (2009). FDG-PET and MRI imaging of the effects of sertindole and haloperidol in the prefrontal lobe in schizophrenia. *Schizophr Res,* 114(1-3), 161-171.

Buchsbaum, M. S., Schoenknecht, P., Torosjan, Y., Newmark, R., Chu, K. W., Mitelman, S., et al. (2006). Diffusion tensor imaging of frontal lobe white matter tracts in schizophrenia. *Ann Gen Psychiatry,* 5, 19.

Buckley, M. J. (2005). The role of the perirhinal cortex and hippocampus in learning, memory and perception. *The Quarterly Journal of Experimental Psychology,* 58(B), 246-268.

Buckley, P. F. (2006). Prevalence and consequences of the dual diagnosis of substance abuse and severe mental illness. *J Clin Psychiatry,* 67 Suppl 7, 5-9.

Burgess, A. P., & Gruzelier, J. H. (1997). Short duration synchronization of human theta rhythm during recognition memory. *Neuroreport,* 8(4), 1039-1042.

Burgess, P. W., Dumontheil, I., & Gilbert, S. J. (2007). The gateway hypothesis of rostral prefrontal cortex (area 10) function. *Trends Cogn Sci,* 11(7), 290-298.

Burns, M. S., & Fahy, J. (2010). Broca's area: rethinking classical concepts from a neuroscience perspective. *Top Stroke Rehabil,* 17(6), 401-410.

Bush, G. (2008). Neuroimaging of attention deficit hyperactivity disorder: can new imaging findings be integrated in clinical practice? *Child Adolesc Psychiatr Clin N Am,* 17(2), 385-404

Bush, G., Frazier, J. A., Rauch, S. L., Seidman, L. J., Whalen, P. J., Jenike, M. A., et al. (1999). Anterior cingulate cortex dysfunction in attention-deficit/hyperactivity disorder revealed by fMRI and the Counting Stroop. *Biol Psychiatry,* 45(12), 1542-1552.

Bush, G., Luu, P., & Posner, M. I. (2000). Cognitive and emotional influences in anterior cingulate cortex. *Trends Cogn Sci,* 4(6), 215-222.

Bush, G., & Shin, L. M. (2006). The Multi-Source Interference Task: an fMRI task that reliably activates the cingulo-frontal-parietal cognitive/attention network. *Nat Protoc,* 1(1), 308-313.

Bush, G., Spencer, T. J., Holmes, J., Shin, L. M., Valera, E. M., Seidman, L. J., et al. (2008). Functional magnetic resonance imaging of methylphenidate and placebo in attention-deficit/hyperactivity disorder during the multi-source interference task. *Arch Gen Psychiatry,* 65(1), 102-114.

Bush, G., Valera, E. M., & Seidman, L. J. (2005). Functional neuroimaging of attention-deficit/ hyperactivity disorder: a review and suggested future directions. *Biol Psychiatry*, 57(11), 1273-1284.

Bush, G., Vogt, B. A., Holmes, J., Dale, A. M., Greve, D., Jenike, M. A., et al. (2002). Dorsal anterior cingulate cortex: a role in reward-based decision making. *Proc Natl Acad Sci U S A*, 99(1), 523-528.

Bushara, K. O., Hanakawa, T., Immisch, I., Toma, K., Kansaku, K., & Hallett, M. (2003). Neural correlates of cross-modal binding. *Nat Neurosci*, 6(2), 190-195.

Buss, K. A., Schumacher, J. R., Dolski, I., Kalin, N. H., Goldsmith, H. H., & Davidson, R. J. (2003). Right frontal brain activity, cortisol, and withdrawal behavior in 6-month-old infants. *Behav Neurosci*, 117(1), 11-20.

Butcher, J. (2001). Self-image contained within right frontal lobe. *Lancet,* 357(9267), 1505.

Cabeza, R., Dolcos, F., Prince, S. E., Rice, H. J., Weissman, D. H., & Nyberg, L. (2003). Attention-related activity during episodic memory retrieval: a cross-function fMRI study. *Neuropsychologia,* 41(3), 390-399.

Cabeza, R., Locantore, J. K., & Anderson, N. D. (2003). Lateralization of prefrontal activity during episodic memory retrieval: evidence for the production-monitoring hypothesis. *J Cogn Neurosci*, 15(2), 249-259.

Cabeza, R., & Nyberg, L. (2000). Imaging cognition II: An empirical review of 275 PET and fMRI studies. *J Cogn Neurosci*, 12(1), 1-47.

Cabeza, R., & Nyberg, L. (2003). Functional neuroimaging of memory. *Neuropsychologia*, 41(3), 241-244.

Cabeza, R., Prince, S. E., Daselaar, S. M., Greenberg, D. L., Budde, M., Dolcos, F., et al. (2004). Brain activity during episodic retrieval of autobiographical and laboratory events: an fMRI study using a novel photo paradigm. *J Cogn Neurosci*, 16(9), 1583-1594.

Caetano, S. C., Fonseca, M., Hatch, J. P., Olvera, R. L., Nicoletti, M., Hunter, K., et al. (2007). Medial temporal lobe abnormalities in pediatric unipolar depression. *Neurosci Lett*, 427(3), 142-147.

Calder, A. J. (2003). Disgust discussed. *Ann Neurol*, 53(4), 427-428.

Call, J., & Tomasello, M. (2008). Does the chimpanzee have a theory of mind? 30 years later. Trends Cogn Sci, 12(5), 187-192.

Cannon, R. (2007). *The effects of spatial-specific neurofeedback training in anterior cingulate cortex*. University of Tennessee, Knoxville.

Cannon, R. (2009). *Functional connectivity in cortical core components of the self and the default network of the brain*. Unpublished Dissertation, Tennessee, Knoxville.

Cannon, R., Baldwin, D. & Lubar, J. (2008). Self-perception and experiential schemata in the addicted brain. *Appl Psychophysiol Biofeedback*, 33(4), 223-238.

Cannon, R., Congedo, M., Lubar, J., & Hutchens, T. (2009). Differentiating a network of executive attention: LORETA neurofeedback in anterior cingulate and dorsolateral prefrontal cortices. *Int J Neurosci*, 119(3), 404-441.

Cannon, R., Congedo, M., Lubar, J., Hutchens, T. (2009). Differentiating at network of executive attention: LORETA Neurofeedback in anterior cingulate and dorsolateral prefrontal cortices. [original research]. *International Journal of Neuroscience*, 119(3), 404 - 441.

Cannon, R., & Lubar, J. (2008). EEG Spectral Power and Coherence: Differentiating Effects of Spatial-Specific Neuro-Operant Learning (SSNOL) Utilizing LORETA Neurofeedback Training in the Anterior Cingulate and Bilateral Dorsolateral Prefrontal Cortices. *Journal of Neurotherapy: Investigations in Neuromodulation, Neurofeedback and Applied Neuroscience*, 11(3), 25 - 44.

Cannon, R., Lubar, J., & Baldwin, D. (2008). Self-perception and experiential schemata in the addicted brain. *Appl Psychophysiol Biofeedback*, 33(4), 223-238.

Cannon, R., Lubar, J., Congedo, M., Thornton, K., Towler, K., & Hutchens, T. (2007). The effects of neurofeedback training in the cognitive division of the anterior cingulate gyrus. *Int J Neurosci*, 117(3), 337-357.

Cannon, R., Lubar, J., Gerke, A., Thornton, K., Hutchens, T., & McCammon, V. (2006). EEG Spectral-Power and Coherence: LORETA Neurofeedback Training in the Anterior Cingulate Gyrus. *Journal of Neurotherapy: Investigations in Neuromodulation, Neurofeedback and Applied Neuroscience*, 10(1), 5 - 31.

Cannon, R., Lubar, J., Sokhadze, E., & Baldwin, D. (2008). LORETA Neurofeedback for Addiction and the Possible Neurophysiology of Psychological Processes Influenced: A Case Study and Region of Interest Analysis of LORETA Neurofeedback in Right Anterior Cingulate Cortex. *Journal of Neurotherapy: Investigations in Neuromodulation, Neurofeedback and Applied Neuroscience*, 12(4), 227 - 241.

Cannon, R., Lubar, J., Thornton, K., Wilson, S., & Congedo, M. (2005). Limbic Beta Activation and LORETA: Can Hippocampal and Related Limbic Activity Be Recorded and Changes Visualized Using LORETA in an Affective Memory Condition? *Journal of Neurotherapy: Investigations in Neuromodulation, Neurofeedback and Applied Neuroscience*, 8(4), 5 - 24.

Cannon, R., Lubar, J (2008). Spectral Power and Coherence: Differentiating effects of Spatial-Specific Neuro-Operant Learning (SSNOL) Utilizing LORETA Neurofeedback Training in the anterior cingulate and bilateral dorsolateral prefrontal cortices. *Journal of Neurotherapy*, 11(3), 25 - 44.

Cannon, R., Lubar, J., Clements, J.G., Harvey, E., Baldwin, D. (2008). Practical Joking and Cingulate Cortex: A Standardized Low-Resolution Electromagnetic Tomography (sLORETA) Investigation of Practical Joking in the Cerebral Volume. *Journal of Neurotherapy* 11(4), 51 - 63.

Cannon, R., Lubar, J., Gerke, A., Thornton, K., Hutchens, T., McCammon, V (2006). Topographical coherence and absolute power changes resulting from LORETA Neurofeedback in the anterior cingulate gyrus. [original research]. *Journal of Neurotherapy*, 10(1), 5 - 31.

Cannon, R., Lubar, J., Thornton, K., Wilson, S., Congedo, M (2004). Limbic Beta Activation and LORETA: Can Hippocampal and Related Limbic Activity Be Recorded And Changes Visualized In An Affective Memory Condition? *Journal of Neurotherapy* 8(4), 5 - 24.

Cannon, R., Lubar, J., Thornton, K., Wilson, S., Congedo, M (2005). Limbic Beta Activation and LORETA: Can Hippocampal and Related Limbic Activity Be Recorded And Changes Visualized In An Affective Memory Condition? *Journal of Neurotherapy* 8(4), 5 - 24.

Cannon, R., Sokhadze, E., Lubar, J., Baldwin, D. (2008). LORETA Neurofeedback for Addiction and the Possible Neurophysiology of Psychological Processes Influenced: A Case Study and Region of Interest Analysis of LORETA Neurofeedback in Right Anterior Cingulate Cortex. *Journal of Neurotherapy*, 12(4), 227 - 241.

Cannon, R., Thatcher, R.W., Lubar, J.F, Baldwin, D.R. (2009). EEG LORETA and the Default Network of Brain. *Paper presented at the Human Behavior-Computational Intelligence Modeling and Interoperability*: Proceedings of the First Conference, Oak Ridge National Laboratory.

Cannon, R. L. (2009). *Functional Connectivity of EEG LORETA in core coponents of the self and the default network (DNt) of the brain.* Unpublished Dissertation, University of Tennessee, Knoxville.

Cannon, R. L., Baldwin, D.R., Lubar, J.F. (2009). Self, Other and Object Processing in the Addicted Brain. In Conference Presentations at the 2009 International Society for Neurofeedback and Research (ISNR) 17th Annual Conference, Indianapolis, Indiana. *Journal of Neurotherapy: Investigations in Neuromodulation, Neurofeedback and Applied Neuroscience*, 13(4), 239 - 276.

Cardinal, R. N., Parkinson, J. A., Hall, J., & Everitt, B. J. (2002). Emotion and motivation: the role of the amygdala, ventral striatum, and prefrontal cortex. *Neurosci Biobehav Rev*, 26(3), 321-352.

Carmona, S., Vilarroya, O., Bielsa, A., Tremols, V., Soliva, J. C., Rovira, M., et al. (2005). Global and regional gray matter reductions in ADHD: a voxel-based morphometric study. *Neurosci Lett*, 389(2), 88-93.

Casanova, M. F., Switala, A. E., & Trippe, J. (2007). A comparison study of the vertical bias of pyramidal cells in the hippocampus and neocortex. *Dev Neurosci*, 29(1-2), 193-200.

Castellanos, F. X. (2001). Neural substrates of attention-deficit hyperactivity disorder. *Adv Neurol*, 85, 197-206.

Castellanos, F. X., & Acosta, M. T. (2002). [Syndrome of attention deficit with hyperactivity as the expression of an organic functional disorder]. *Rev Neurol*, 35(1), 1-11.

Castellanos, F. X., Giedd, J. N., Marsh, W. L., Hamburger, S. D., Vaituzis, A. C., Dickstein, D. P., et al. (1996). Quantitative brain magnetic resonance imaging in attention-deficit hyperactivity disorder. *Arch Gen Psychiatry*, 53(7), 607-616.

Castellanos, F. X., Glaser, P. E., & Gerhardt, G. A. (2006). Towards a neuroscience of attention-deficit/hyperactivity disorder: fractionating the phenotype. *J Neurosci Methods,* 151(1), 1-4.

Castellanos, F. X., Margulies, D. S., Kelly, C., Uddin, L. Q., Ghaffari, M., Kirsch, A., et al. (2008). Cingulate-precuneus interactions: a new locus of dysfunction in adult attention-deficit/hyperactivity disorder. *Biol Psychiatry*, 63(3), 332-337.

Castellanos, F. X., Sharp, W. S., Gottesman, R. F., Greenstein, D. K., Giedd, J. N., & Rapoport, J. L. (2003). Anatomic brain abnormalities in monozygotic twins discordant for attention deficit hyperactivity disorder. *Am J Psychiatry*, 160(9), 1693-1696.

Castellanos, F. X., & Tannock, R. (2002). Neuroscience of attention-deficit/hyperactivity disorder: the search for endophenotypes. *Nat Rev Neurosci*, 3(8), 617-628.

Cavanna, A. E., & Trimble, M. R. (2006). The precuneus: a review of its functional anatomy and behavioural correlates. *Brain*, 129(Pt 3), 564-583.

Chakravorty, N. K. (1982). Parietal lobe syndrome due to cerebrovascular accidents. *Practitioner*, 226(1363), 129-131.

Chana, G., Landau, S., Beasley, C., Everall, I. P., & Cotter, D. (2003). Two-dimensional assessment of cytoarchitecture in the anterior cingulate cortex in major depressive disorder, bipolar disorder, and schizophrenia: evidence for decreased neuronal somal size and increased neuronal density. *Biol Psychiatry*, 53(12), 1086-1098.

Chen, W., Tenney, J., Kulkarni, P., & King, J. A. (2007). Imaging unconditioned fear response with manganese-enhanced MRI (MEMRI). *Neuroimage*, 37(1), 221-229.

Choi, J., Jeong, B., Rohan, M. L., Polcari, A. M., & Teicher, M. H. (2009). Preliminary evidence for white matter tract abnormalities in young adults exposed to parental verbal abuse. *Biol Psychiatry*, 65(3), 227-234.

Choo, I. H., Lee, D. Y., Oh, J. S., Lee, J. S., Lee, D. S., Song, I. C., et al. (2008). Posterior cingulate cortex atrophy and regional cingulum disruption in mild cognitive impairment and Alzheimer's disease. *Neurobiol Aging*. 31:772-779

Chow, C. C., & Kopell, N. (2000). Dynamics of spiking neurons with electrical coupling. *Neural Comput*, 12(7), 1643-1678.

Chow, K. L., & Hutt, P. J. (1953). The association cortex of Macaca mulatta: a review of recent contributions to its anatomy and functions. *Brain*, 76(4), 625-677.

Christodoulou, C., DeLuca, J., Ricker, J., Madigan, N., Bly, B., Lange, G., et al. (2001). Functional magnetic resonance imaging of working memory impairment following traumatic brain injury. *J Neurol Neurosurg Psychi*. 71:161-168

Chugani, H. T., Muller, R. A., & Chugani, D. C. (1996). Functional brain reorganization in children. *Brain Dev*, 18(5), 347-356.

Cicchetti, D., & Rogosch, F. A. (1997). The role of self-organization in the promotion of resilience in maltreated children. *Dev Psychopathol*, 9(4), 797-815.

Clarke, A. R., Barry, R. J., McCarthy, R., Selikowitz, M., Johnstone, S. J., Hsu, C. I., et al. (2007). Coherence in children with Attention-Deficit/Hyperactivity Disorder and excess beta activity in their EEG. *Clin Neurophysiol*, 118(7), 1472-1479.

Clerget, E., Winderickx, A., Fadiga, L., & Olivier, E. (2009). Role of Broca's area in encoding sequential human actions: a virtual lesion study. *Neuroreport*, 20(16), 1496-1499.

Clugnet, M. C., & LeDoux, J. E. (1990). Synaptic plasticity in fear conditioning circuits: induction of LTP in the lateral nucleus of the amygdala by stimulation of the medial geniculate body. *J Neurosci,* 10(8), 2818-2824.

Clugnet, M. C., LeDoux, J. E., & Morrison, S. F. (1990). Unit responses evoked in the amygdala and striatum by electrical stimulation of the medial geniculate body. *J Neurosci*, 10(4), 1055-1061.

Coburn, K. L., Lauterbach, E. C., Boutros, N. N., Black, K. J., Arciniegas, D. B., & Coffey, C. E. (2006). The value of quantitative electroencephalography in clinical psychiatry: a report by the Committee on Research of the American Neuropsychiatric Association. *J Neuropsychiatry Clin Neurosci,* 18(4), 460-500.

Cohen, D., Cuffin, B. N., Yunokuchi, K., Maniewski, R., Purcell, C., Cosgrove, G. R., et al. (1990). MEG versus EEG localization test using implanted sources in the human brain. *Ann Neurol*, 28(6), 811-817.

Cohen, D. A., Prud'homme, M. J., & Kalaska, J. F. (1994). Tactile activity in primate primary somatosensory cortex during active arm movements: correlation with receptive field properties. *J Neurophysiol*, 71(1), 161-172.

Colla, M., Ende, G., Alm, B., Deuschle, M., Heuser, I., & Kronenberg, G. (2008). Cognitive MR spectroscopy of anterior cingulate cortex in ADHD: elevated choline signal correlates with slowed hit reaction times. *J Psychiatr Res*, 42(7), 587-595.

Congedo, M. (2003). *Tomographic neurofeedback: a new technique for the self-regulation of brain electrical activity.* Unpublished Dissertation, Tennessee, Knoxville.

Congedo, M. (2006). Subspace projection filters for real-time brain electromagnetic imaging. *IEEE Trans Biomed Eng*, 53(8), 1624-1634.

Congedo, M., Lotte, F., & Lecuyer, A. (2006). Classification of movement intention by spatially filtered electromagnetic inverse solutions. *Phys Med Biol*, 51(8), 1971-1989.

Congedo, M., Lubar, J. F., & Joffe, D. (2004). Low-resolution electromagnetic tomography neurofeedback. *IEEE Trans Neural Syst Rehabil Eng*, 12(4), 387-397.

Connemann, B. J., Mann, K., Lange-Asschenfeldt, C., Ruchsow, M., Schreckenberger, M., Bartenstein, P., et al. (2005). Anterior limbic alpha-like activity: a low resolution electromagnetic tomography study with lorazepam challenge. *Clin Neurophysiol*, 116(4), 886-894.

Conway, M. A., Pleydell-Pearce, C. W., Whitecross, S. E., & Sharpe, H. (2003). Neurophysiological correlates of memory for experienced and imagined events. *Neuropsychologia*, 41(3), 334-340.

Cook, B. L., Shukla, S., & Hoff, A. L. (1986). EEG abnormalities in bipolar affective disorder. *J Affect Disord*, 11(2), 147-149.

Corbetta, M., Akbudak, E., Conturo, T. E., Snyder, A. Z., Ollinger, J. M., Drury, H. A., et al. (1998). A common network of functional areas for attention and eye movements. *Neuron*, 21(4), 761-773.

Corsi-Cabrera, M., Galindo-Vilchis, L., del-Rio-Portilla, Y., Arce, C., & Ramos-Loyo, J. (2007). Within-subject reliability and inter-session stability of EEG power and coherent activity in women evaluated monthly over nine months. *Clin Neurophysiol*, 118(1), 9-21.

Corsi-Cabrera, M., Guevara, M. A., Arce, C., & Ramos, J. (1996). Inter and intrahemispheric EEG correlation as a function of sleep cycles. *Prog Neuropsychopharmacol Biol Psychiatry*, 20(3), 387-405.

Corsi-Cabrera, M., Solis-Ortiz, S., & Guevara, M. A. (1997). Stability of EEG inter- and intrahemispheric correlation in women. *Electroencephalogr Clin Neurophysiol*, 102(3), 248-255.

Cotter, D., Landau, S., Beasley, C., Stevenson, R., Chana, G., MacMillan, L., et al. (2002). The density and spatial distribution of GABAergic neurons, labelled using calcium binding proteins, in the anterior cingulate cortex in major depressive disorder, bipolar disorder, and schizophrenia. *Biol Psychiatry*, 51(5), 377-386.

Cottler, L. B., Compton, W. M., 3rd, Mager, D., Spitznagel, E. L., & Janca, A. (1992). Posttraumatic stress disorder among substance users from the general population. *Am J Psychiatry*, 149(5), 664-670.

Coutin-Churchman, P., Anez, Y., Uzcategui, M., Alvarez, L., Vergara, F., Mendez, L., et al. (2003). Quantitative spectral analysis of EEG in psychiatry revisited: drawing signs out of numbers in a clinical setting. *Clin Neurophysiol*, 114(12), 2294-2306.

Coutin-Churchman, P., & Moreno, R. (2008). Intracranial current density (LORETA) differences in QEEG frequency bands between depressed and non-depressed alcoholic patients. *Clin Neurophysiol*, 119(4), 948-958.

Coutin-Churchman, P., Moreno, R., Anez, Y., & Vergara, F. (2006). Clinical correlates of quantitative EEG alterations in alcoholic patients. *Clin Neurophysiol*, 117(4), 740-751.

Craig, A. D. (2009a). Emotional moments across time: a possible neural basis for time perception in the anterior insula. *Philos Trans R Soc Lond B Biol Sci*, 364(1525), 1933-1942.

Craig, A. D. (2009b). How do you feel--now? The anterior insula and human awareness. Nat Rev Neurosci, 10(1), 59-70.

Critchley, H. D. (2005). Neural mechanisms of autonomic, affective, and cognitive integration. *J Comp Neurol*, 493(1), 154-166.

Critchley, H. D., Daly, E. M., Bullmore, E. T., Williams, S. C., Van Amelsvoort, T., Robertson, D. M., et al. (2000). The functional neuroanatomy of social behaviour: changes in cerebral blood flow when people with autistic disorder process facial expressions. *Brain*, 123 (Pt 11), 2203-2212.

Critchley, H. D., Elliott, R., Mathias, C. J., & Dolan, R. J. (2000). Neural activity relating to generation and representation of galvanic skin conductance responses: a functional magnetic resonance imaging study. *J Neurosci*, 20(8), 3033-3040.

Critchley, H. D., Mathias, C. J., Josephs, O., O'Doherty, J., Zanini, S., Dewar, B. K., et al. (2003). Human cingulate cortex and autonomic control: converging neuroimaging and clinical evidence. *Brain*, 126(Pt 10), 2139-2152.

Cummings, J. L. (1997). Neuropsychiatric manifestations of right hemisphere lesions. *Brain Lang*, 57(1), 22-37.

Czobor, P., & Volavka, J. (1991). Pretreatment EEG predicts short-term response to haloperidol treatment. *Biol Psychiatry*, 30(9), 927-942.

D'Angiulli, A., Grunau, P., Maggi, S., & Herdman, A. (2006). Electroencephalographic correlates of prenatal exposure to alcohol in infants and children: a review of findings and implications for neurocognitive development. *Alcohol*, 40(2), 127-133.

Dagher, A., Tannenbaum, B., Hayashi, T., Pruessner, J. C., & McBride, D. (2009). An acute psychosocial stress enhances the neural response to smoking cues. *Brain Res*, 1293, 40-48.

Dalton, K. M., Kalin, N. H., Grist, T. M., & Davidson, R. J. (2005). Neural-cardiac coupling in threat-evoked anxiety. *J Cogn Neurosci*, 17(6), 969-980.

Damasio, A. R., & Geschwind, N. (1984). The neural basis of language. *Annu Rev Neurosci, 7*, 127-147.

Damasio, A. R., Grabowski, T. J., Bechara, A., Damasio, H., Ponto, L. L., Parvizi, J., et al. (2000). Subcortical and cortical brain activity during the feeling of self-generated emotions. *Nat Neurosci*, 3(10), 1049-1056.

Damoiseaux, J. S., Beckmann, C. F., Arigita, E. J., Barkhof, F., Scheltens, P., Stam, C. J., et al. (2008). Reduced resting-state brain activity in the "default network" in normal aging. *Cereb Cortex*, 18(8), 1856-1864.

Damoiseaux, J. S., Rombouts, S. A., Barkhof, F., Scheltens, P., Stam, C. J., Smith, S. M., et al. (2006). Consistent resting-state networks across healthy subjects. *Proc Natl Acad Sci U S A*, 103(37), 13848-13853.

Dardou, D., Datiche, F., & Cattarelli, M. (2007). Does taste or odor activate the same brain networks after retrieval of taste potentiated odor aversion? *Neurobiol Learn Mem*, 88(2), 186-197.

Davidson, R. J. (2000). Affective style, psychopathology, and resilience: brain mechanisms and plasticity. *Am Psychol*, 55(11), 1196-1214.

Davidson, R. J. (2002). Anxiety and affective style: role of prefrontal cortex and amygdala. *Biol Psychiatry*, 51(1), 68-80.

Davidson, R. J. (2004). What does the prefrontal cortex "do" in affect: perspectives on frontal EEG asymmetry research. *Biol Psychol*, 67(1-2), 219-233.

Davidson, R. J., Coe, C. C., Dolski, I., & Donzella, B. (1999). Individual differences in prefrontal activation asymmetry predict natural killer cell activity at rest and in response to challenge. *Brain Behav Immun*, 13(2), 93-108.

Davidson, R. J., & Irwin, W. (1999). The functional neuroanatomy of emotion and affective style. *Trends Cogn Sci*, 3(1), 11-21.

Davidson, R. J., Irwin, W., Anderle, M. J., & Kalin, N. H. (2003). The neural substrates of affective processing in depressed patients treated with venlafaxine. *Am J Psychiatry*, 160(1), 64-75.

Davidson, R. J., Jackson, D. C., & Kalin, N. H. (2000). Emotion, plasticity, context, and regulation: perspectives from affective neuroscience. *Psychol Bull*, 126(6), 890-909.

Davidson, R. J., Kalin, N. H., & Shelton, S. E. (1993). Lateralized response to diazepam predicts temperamental style in rhesus monkeys. *Behav Neurosci*, 107(6), 1106-1110.

Davidson, R. J., Pizzagalli, D., Nitschke, J. B., & Putnam, K. (2002). Depression: perspectives from affective neuroscience. *Annu Rev Psychol*, 53, 545-574.

Davidson, R. J., Putnam, K. M., & Larson, C. L. (2000). Dysfunction in the neural circuitry of emotion regulation--a possible prelude to violence. *Science*, 289(5479), 591-594.

Davidson, R. J., & Slagter, H. A. (2000). Probing emotion in the developing brain: functional neuroimaging in the assessment of the neural substrates of emotion in normal and disordered children and adolescents. *Ment Retard Dev Disabil Res Rev*, 6(3), 166-170.

Dawson, G., Panagiotides, H., Klinger, L. G., & Spieker, S. (1997). Infants of depressed and nondepressed mothers exhibit differences in frontal brain electrical activity during the expression of negative emotions. *Dev Psychol*, 33(4), 650-656.

de Greck, M., Rotte, M., Paus, R., Moritz, D., Thiemann, R., Proesch, U., et al. (2008). Is our self based on reward? Self-relatedness recruits neural activity in the reward system. *Neuroimage*, 39(4), 2066-2075.

De Luca, M., Beckmann, C. F., De Stefano, N., Matthews, P. M., & Smith, S. M. (2006). fMRI resting state networks define distinct modes of long-distance interactions in the human brain. *Neuroimage,* 29(4), 1359-1367.

De Ridder, D., Van Laere, K., Dupont, P., Menovsky, T., & Van de Heyning, P. (2007). Visualizing out-of-body experience in the brain. *N Engl J Med*, 357(18), 1829-1833.

de Vries, M. H., Barth, A. C., Maiworm, S., Knecht, S., Zwitserlood, P., & Floel, A. (2010). Electrical stimulation of Broca's area enhances implicit learning of an artificial grammar. *J Cogn Neurosci*, 22(11), 2427-2436.

DeBruine, L. M. (2004). Facial resemblance increases the attractiveness of same-sex faces more than other-sex faces. *Proc Biol Sci*, 271(1552), 2085-2090.

Dedovic, K., Duchesne, A., Andrews, J., Engert, V., & Pruessner, J. C. (2009). The brain and the stress axis: the neural correlates of cortisol regulation in response to stress. *Neuroimage*, 47(3), 864-871.

Dedovic, K., Renwick, R., Mahani, N. K., Engert, V., Lupien, S. J., & Pruessner, J. C. (2005). The Montreal Imaging Stress Task: using functional imaging to investigate the effects of perceiving and processing psychosocial stress in the human brain. *J Psychiatry Neurosci*, 30(5), 319-325.

Dehaene, S., & Changeux, J. P. (2000). Reward-dependent learning in neuronal networks for planning and decision making. *Prog Brain Res*, 126, 217-229.

del Olmo, N., Miguens, M., Higuera-Matas, A., Torres, I., Garcia-Lecumberri, C., Solis, J. M., et al. (2006). Enhancement of hippocampal long-term potentiation induced by cocaine self-administration is maintained during the extinction of this behavior. *Brain Res*, 1116(1), 120-126.

Delgado, M. R., Miller, M. M., Inati, S., & Phelps, E. A. (2005). An fMRI study of reward-related probability learning. *Neuroimage*, 24(3), 862-873.

Deppe, M., Schwindt, W., Kugel, H., Plassmann, H., & Kenning, P. (2005). Nonlinear responses within the medial prefrontal cortex reveal when specific implicit information influences economic decision making. *J Neuroimaging*, 15(2), 171-182.

Dettling, A. C., Gunnar, M. R., & Donzella, B. (1999). Cortisol levels of young children in full-day childcare centers: relations with age and temperament. *Psychoneuroendocrinology*, 24(5), 519-536.

Deutschlander, A., Bense, S., Stephan, T., Schwaiger, M., Brandt, T., & Dieterich, M. (2002). Sensory system interactions during simultaneous vestibular and visual stimulation in PET. *Hum Brain Mapp*, 16(2), 92-103.

Devinsky, O., Morrell, M. J., & Vogt, B. A. (1995). Contributions of anterior cingulate cortex to behaviour. *Brain*, 118 (Pt 1), 279-306.

Dewan, M. J., Haldipur, C. V., Boucher, M. F., Ramachandran, T., & Major, L. F. (1988). Bipolar affective disorder. II. EEG, neuropsychological, and clinical correlates of CT abnormality. *Acta Psychiatr Scand*, 77(6), 677-682.

Di Chiara, G. (1995). The role of dopamine in drug abuse viewed from the perspective of its role in motivation. *Drug Alcohol Depend*, 38(2), 95-137.

Di Chiara, G., Tanda, G., Bassareo, V., Pontieri, F., Acquas, E., Fenu, S., et al. (1999). Drug addiction as a disorder of associative learning. Role of nucleus accumbens shell/extended amygdala dopamine. *Ann N Y Acad Sci,* 877, 461-485.

Diamond, D. M., Campbell, A. M., Park, C. R., Halonen, J., & Zoladz, P. R. (2007). The temporal dynamics model of emotional memory processing: a synthesis on the neurobiological basis of stress-induced amnesia, flashbulb and traumatic memories, and the Yerkes-Dodson law. *Neural Plast*, 60803.

Dickerson, S. S., & Kemeny, M. E. (2004). Acute stressors and cortisol responses: a theoretical integration and synthesis of laboratory research. *Psychol Bull,* 130(3), 355-391.

Dienstbier, R. A., Hillman, D., Lehnhoff, J., Hillman, J., & Valkenaar, M. C. (1975). An emotion-attribution approach to moral behavior: interfacing cognitive and avoidance theories of moral development. *Psychol Rev,* 82(4), 299-315.

Doppelmayr, M., Klimesch, W., Hodlmoser, K., Sauseng, P., & Gruber, W. (2005). Intelligence related upper alpha desynchronization in a semantic memory task. *Brain Res Bull,* 66(2), 171-177.

Doppelmayr, M., Klimesch, W., Sauseng, P., Hodlmoser, K., Stadler, W., & Hanslmayr, S. (2005). Intelligence related differences in EEG-bandpower. *Neurosci Lett*, 381(3), 309-313.

Downey, K. K., Stelson, F. W., Pomerleau, O. F., & Giordani, B. (1997). Adult attention deficit hyperactivity disorder: psychological test profiles in a clinical population. *J Nerv Ment Dis*, 185(1), 32-38.

Drake, R. E., & Wallach, M. A. (2000). Dual diagnosis: 15 years of progress. *Psychiatr Serv*, 51(9), 1126-1129.

Drevets, W. C. (2007). Orbitofrontal Cortex Function and Structure in Depression. *Ann N Y Acad Sci.* 1121:499-527

Drevets, W. C., Gautier, C., Price, J. C., Kupfer, D. J., Kinahan, P. E., Grace, A. A., et al. (2001). Amphetamine-induced dopamine release in human ventral striatum correlates with euphoria. *Biol Psychiatry*, 49(2), 81-96.

du Boisgueheneuc, F., Levy, R., Volle, E., Seassau, M., Duffau, H., Kinkingnehun, S., et al. (2006). Functions of the left superior frontal gyrus in humans: a lesion study. *Brain*, 129(Pt 12), 3315-3328.

Dual diagnosis. Part II. A look at old reliable and promising new approaches to the treatment of mental illness with substance abuse (2003). *Harv Ment Health Lett,* 20(3), 1-5.

Dual diagnosis: Part I. Mental illness and substance abuse can be a devastating combination, but help is increasingly available (2003). *Harv Ment Health Lett*, 20(2), 1-4.

Dudukovic, N. M., & Wagner, A. D. (2007). Goal-dependent modulation of declarative memory: neural correlates of temporal recency decisions and novelty detection. *Neuropsychologia*, 45(11), 2608-2620.

Dupont, S. (2002). Investigating temporal pole function by functional imaging. *Epileptic Disord*, 4 Suppl 1, S17-22.

Durka, P. J., Klekowicz, H., Blinowska, K. J., Szelenberger, W., & Niemcewicz, S. (2003). A simple system for detection of EEG artifacts in polysomnographic recordings. *IEEE Trans Biomed Eng*, 50(4), 526-528.

Durston, S. (2003). A review of the biological bases of ADHD: what have we learned from imaging studies? *Ment Retard Dev Disabil Res Rev*, 9(3), 184-195.

Durston, S., Tottenham, N. T., Thomas, K. M., Davidson, M. C., Eigsti, I. M., Yang, Y., et al. (2003). Differential patterns of striatal activation in young children with and without ADHD. *Biol Psychiatry*, 53(10), 871-878.

Egger, M. D., & Flynn, J. P. (1962). Amygdaloid suppression of hypothalamically elicited attack behavior. *Science*, 136, 43-44.

Egloff, B., Schmukle, S. C., Burns, L. R., & Schwerdtfeger, A. (2006). Spontaneous emotion regulation during evaluated speaking tasks: associations with negative affect, anxiety expression, memory, and physiological responding. *Emotion*, 6(3), 356-366.

Elbert, T., Lutzenberger, W., Rockstroh, B., & Birbaumer, N. (1985). Removal of ocular artifacts from the EEG--a biophysical approach to the EOG. *Electroencephalogr Clin Neurophysiol*, 60(5), 455-463.

Enzi, B., de Greck, M., Prosch, U., Tempelmann, C., & Northoff, G. (2009). Is our self nothing but reward? Neuronal overlap and distinction between reward and personal relevance and its relation to human personality. *PLoS One*, 4(12), e8429.

Essl, M., & Rappelsberger, P. (1998). EEG coherence and reference signals: experimental results and mathematical explanations. *Med Biol Eng Comput*, 36(4), 399-406.

Esslen, M., Pascual-Marqui, R. D., Hell, D., Kochi, K., & Lehmann, D. (2004). Brain areas and time course of emotional processing. *Neuroimage*, 21(4), 1189-1203.

Evans, K. C., Wright, C. I., Wedig, M. M., Gold, A. L., Pollack, M. H., & Rauch, S. L. (2007). A functional MRI study of amygdala responses to angry schematic faces in social anxiety disorder. *Depress Anxiety*. 25:496-505

Fair, D. A., Cohen, A. L., Dosenbach, N. U., Church, J. A., Miezin, F. M., Barch, D. M., et al. (2008). The maturing architecture of the brain's default network. *Proc Natl Acad Sci U S A*, 105(10), 4028-4032.

Fair, D. A., Posner, J., Nagel, B. J., Bathula, D., Dias, T. G., Mills, K. L., et al. (2010a). Atypical default network connectivity in youth with attention-deficit/hyperactivity disorder. *Biol Psychiatry*, 68(12), 1084-1091.

Fair, D. A., Posner, J., Nagel, B. J., Bathula, D., Dias, T. G., Mills, K. L., et al. (2010b). Atypical Default Network Connectivity in Youth with Attention-Deficit/Hyperactivity Disorder. *Biol Psychiatry.*

Faraone, S. V., Biederman, J., & Mick, E. (2006). The age-dependent decline of attention deficit hyperactivity disorder: a meta-analysis of follow-up studies. *Psychol Med*, 36(2), 159-165.

Fein, G., Di Sclafani, V., & Meyerhoff, D. J. (2002). Prefrontal cortical volume reduction associated with frontal cortex function deficit in 6-week abstinent crack-cocaine dependent men. *Drug Alcohol Depend*, 68(1), 87-93.

Fein, G., Raz, J., Brown, F. F., & Merrin, E. L. (1988). Common reference coherence data are confounded by power and phase effects. *Electroencephalogr Clin Neurophysiol*, 69(6), 581-584.

Feldman, S., & Weidenfeld, J. (1995). Neural mechanisms involved in the corticosteroid feedback effects on the hypothalamo-pituitary-adrenocortical axis. *Prog Neurobiol*, 45(2), 129-141.

Fell, J., Klaver, P., Elfadil, H., Schaller, C., Elger, C. E., & Fernandez, G. (2003). Rhinal-hippocampal theta coherence during declarative memory formation: interaction with gamma synchronization? *Eur J Neurosci*, 17(5), 1082-1088.

Fibiger, H. C., & Phillips, A. G. (1988). Mesocorticolimbic dopamine systems and reward. *Ann N Y Acad Sci*, 537, 206-215.

Figueiredo, H. F., Bodie, B. L., Tauchi, M., Dolgas, C. M., & Herman, J. P. (2003). Stress integration after acute and chronic predator stress: differential activation of central stress circuitry and sensitization of the hypothalamo-pituitary-adrenocortical axis. *Endocrinology*, 144(12), 5249-5258.

Figueiredo, H. F., Bruestle, A., Bodie, B., Dolgas, C. M., & Herman, J. P. (2003). The medial prefrontal cortex differentially regulates stress-induced c-fos expression in the forebrain depending on type of stressor. *Eur J Neurosci*, 18(8), 2357-2364.

Fingelkurts, A. A., Krause, C. M., & Sams, M. (2002). Probability interrelations between pre-/post-stimulus intervals and ERD/ERS during a memory task. *Clin Neurophysiol*, 113(6), 826-843.

Fingelkurts, A. A., Rytsala, H., Suominen, K., Isometsa, E., & Kahkonen, S. (2006). Composition of brain oscillations in ongoing EEG during major depression disorder. *Neurosci Res*, 56(2), 133-144.

Fingelkurts, A. A., Rytsala, H., Suominen, K., Isometsa, E., & Kahkonen, S. (2007). Impaired functional connectivity at EEG alpha and theta frequency bands in major depression. *Hum Brain Mapp*, 28(3), 247-261.

Fink, A., & Neubauer, A. C. (2006). EEG alpha oscillations during the performance of verbal creativity tasks: differential effects of sex and verbal intelligence. *Int J Psychophysiol*, 62(1), 46-53.

Fink, M., & Irwin, P. (1976). Pharmacodynamic analyses using quantitative EEG data. *Psychopharmacol Bull*, 12(4), 55-59.

Finn, P. R., Justus, A., Mazas, C., & Steinmetz, J. E. (1999). Working memory, executive processes and the effects of alcohol on Go/No-Go learning: testing a model of behavioral regulation and impulsivity. *Psychopharmacology (Berl)*, 146(4), 465-472.

Fleck, M. S., Daselaar, S. M., Dobbins, I. G., & Cabeza, R. (2006). Role of prefrontal and anterior cingulate regions in decision-making processes shared by memory and nonmemory tasks. *Cereb Cortex*, 16(11), 1623-1630.

Flor-Henry, P., Lind, J. C., & Koles, Z. J. (2004). A source-imaging (low-resolution electromagnetic tomography) study of the EEGs from unmedicated males with depression. *Psychiatry Res*, 130(2), 191-207.

Bookheimer, S. Y., Bilder, R. M., et al. (2008). Selective corticostriatal dysfunction in schizophrenia: examination of motor and cognitive skill learning. *Neuropsychology*, 22(1), 100-109.

Ford, A., McGregor, K. M., Case, K., Crosson, B., & White, K. D. (2010). Structural connectivity of Broca's area and medial frontal cortex. *Neuroimage*, 52(4), 1230-1237.

Fortgens, C., & De Bruin, M. P. (1983). Removal of eye movement and ECG artifacts from the non-cephalic reference EEG. *Electroencephalogr Clin Neurophysiol*, 56(1), 90-96.

Fortin, A., Ptito, A., Faubert, J., & Ptito, M. (2002). Cortical areas mediating stereopsis in the human brain: a PET study. *Neuroreport*, 13(6), 895-898.

Fox, P. T. (1995). Spatial normalization origins: Objectives, applications, and alternatives. *Hum Brain Mapping*, 3, 161-164.

Fransson, P. (2005). Spontaneous low-frequency BOLD signal fluctuations: an fMRI investigation of the resting-state default mode of brain function hypothesis. *Hum Brain Mapp*, 26(1), 15-29.

Fransson, P. (2006). How default is the default mode of brain function? Further evidence from intrinsic BOLD signal fluctuations. *Neuropsychologia*, 44(14), 2836-2845.

Fransson, P., & Marrelec, G. (2008). The precuneus/posterior cingulate cortex plays a pivotal role in the default mode network: Evidence from a partial correlation network analysis. *Neuroimage*, 42(3), 1178-1184.

Fransson, P., Skiold, B., Horsch, S., Nordell, A., Blennow, M., Lagercrantz, H., et al. (2007). Resting-state networks in the infant brain. *Proc Natl Acad Sci U S A*, 104(39), 15531-15536.

Frei, E., Gamma, A., Pascual-Marqui, R., Lehmann, D., Hell, D., & Vollenweider, F. X. (2001). Localization of MDMA-induced brain activity in healthy volunteers using low resolution brain electromagnetic tomography (LORETA). *Hum Brain Mapp*, 14(3), 152-165.

Frey, B. N., Andreazza, A. C., Nery, F. G., Martins, M. R., Quevedo, J., Soares, J. C., et al. (2007). The role of hippocampus in the pathophysiology of bipolar disorder. *Behav Pharmacol*, 18(5-6), 419-430.

Fricchione, G., & Stefano, G. B. (2005). Placebo neural systems: nitric oxide, morphine and the dopamine brain reward and motivation circuitries. *Med Sci Monit*, 11(5), MS54-65.

Friedman, D., Nessler, D., & Johnson, R., Jr. (2007). Memory encoding and retrieval in the aging brain. *Clin EEG Neurosci*, 38(1), 2-7.

Fries, A., Frey, D., & Pongratz, L. J. (1977). [Anxiety, self perception and cognitive dissonance]. *Arch Psychol (Frankf)*, 129(1), 83-98.

Friston, K. J., Frith, C. D., Liddle, P. F., Dolan, R. J., Lammertsma, A. A., & Frackowiak, R. S. (1990). The relationship between global and local changes in PET scans. *J Cereb Blood Flow Metab*, 10(4), 458-466.

Friston, K. J., Frith, C. D., Liddle, P. F., & Frackowiak, R. S. (1991). Comparing functional (PET) images: the assessment of significant change. *J Cereb Blood Flow Metab*, 11(4), 690-699.

Friston, K. J., Holmes, A. P., Poline, J. B., Grasby, P. J., Williams, S. C., Frackowiak, R. S., et al. (1995). Analysis of fMRI time-series revisited. *Neuroimage*, 2(1), 45-53.

Friston, K. J., Liddle, P. F., Frith, C. D., Hirsch, S. R., & Frackowiak, R. S. (1992). The left medial temporal region and schizophrenia. A PET study. *Brain*, 115 (Pt 2), 367-382.

Frith, C. D., Friston, K., Liddle, P. F., & Frackowiak, R. S. (1991a). Willed action and the prefrontal cortex in man: a study with PET. *Proc Biol Sci*, 244(1311), 241-246.

Frith, C. D., Friston, K. J., Liddle, P. F., & Frackowiak, R. S. (1991b). A PET study of word finding. *Neuropsychologia*, 29(12), 1137-1148.

Frith, C. D., Friston, K. J., Liddle, P. F., & Frackowiak, R. S. (1992). PET imaging and cognition in schizophrenia. *J R Soc Med*, 85(4), 222-224.

Frodl, T., Schaub, A., Banac, S., Charypar, M., Jager, M., Kummler, P., et al. (2006). Reduced hippocampal volume correlates with executive dysfunctioning in major depression. *J Psychiatry Neurosci*, 31(5), 316-323.

Furmark, T., Tillfors, M., Marteinsdottir, I., Fischer, H., Pissiota, A., Langstrom, B., et al. (2002). Common changes in cerebral blood flow in patients with social phobia treated with citalopram or cognitive-behavioral therapy. *Arch Gen Psychiatry*, 59(5), 425-433.

Fuster, J. M. (2000a). Executive frontal functions. *Exp Brain Res*, 133(1), 66-70.

Fuster, J. M. (2000b). Prefrontal neurons in networks of executive memory. *Brain Res Bull*, 52(5), 331-336.

Gainetdinov, R. R., Wetsel, W. C., Jones, S. R., Levin, E. D., Jaber, M., & Caron, M. G. (1999). Role of serotonin in the paradoxical calming effect of psychostimulants on hyperactivity. *Science*, 283(5400), 397-401.

Gara, M. A., Woolfolk, R. L., Cohen, B. D., Goldston, R. B., Allen, L. A., & Novalany, J. (1993). Perception of self and other in major depression. *J Abnorm Psychol*, 102(1), 93-100.

Gardini, S., Cornoldi, C., De Beni, R., & Venneri, A. (2006). Left mediotemporal structures mediate the retrieval of episodic autobiographical mental images. *Neuroimage*, 30(2), 645-655.

Garoutte, B., & Aird, R. B. (1958). Studies on the cortical pacemaker: synchrony and asynchrony of bilaterally recorded alpha and beta activity. *Electroencephalogr Clin Neurophysiol*, 10(2), 259-268.

Gass, P., & Riva, M. A. (2007). CREB, neurogenesis and depression. *Bioessays*, 29(10), 957-961.

Gawryluk, J. R., D'Arcy, R. C., Mazerolle, E. L., Brewer, K. D., & Beyea, S. D. (2010). Functional mapping in the corpus callosum: A 4T fMRI study of white matter. *Neuroimage*. 54-10-15

Gehring, W. J., & Knight, R. T. (2002). Lateral prefrontal damage affects processing selection but not attention switching. *Brain Res Cogn Brain Res*, 13(2), 267-279.

Gendolla, G. H., Abele, A. E., Andrei, A., Spurk, D., & Richter, M. (2005). Negative mood, self-focused attention, and the experience of physical symptoms: the joint impact hypothesis. *Emotion*, 5(2), 131-144.

Gittelman, R., Mannuzza, S., Shenker, R., & Bonagura, N. (1985). Hyperactive boys almost grown up. I. Psychiatric status. *Arch Gen Psychiatry*, 42(10), 937-947.

Gluck, J., & Bluck, S. (2007). Looking back across the life span: a life story account of the reminiscence bump. *Mem Cognit*, 35(8), 1928-1939.

Gneo, S., Natoli, N., Menghini, G., & Galanti, A. (1986). [Self perception and body image evaluation in mastectomized women]. *Minerva Ginecol*, 38(7-8), 553-557.

Goel, V., Grafman, J., Sadato, N., & Hallett, M. (1995). Modeling other minds. *Neuroreport*, 6(13), 1741-1746.

Goldapple, K., Segal, Z., Garson, C., Lau, M., Bieling, P., Kennedy, S., et al. (2004). Modulation of cortical-limbic pathways in major depression: treatment-specific effects of cognitive behavior therapy. *Arch Gen Psychiatry*, 61(1), 34-41.

Goldstein, M. L. (1968). Physiological theories of emotion: a critical historical review from the standpoint of behavior theory. *Psychol Bull*, 69(1), 23-40.

Goldstein, R. Z., Alia-Klein, N., Tomasi, D., Zhang, L., Cottone, L. A., Maloney, T., et al. (2007). Is decreased prefrontal cortical sensitivity to monetary reward associated with impaired motivation and self-control in cocaine addiction? *Am J Psychiatry*, 164(1), 43-51.

Goldstein, R. Z., Tomasi, D., Rajaram, S., Cottone, L. A., Zhang, L., Maloney, T., et al. (2007). Role of the anterior cingulate and medial orbitofrontal cortex in processing drug cues in cocaine addiction. *Neuroscience*, 144(4), 1153-1159.

Gomez, J. F., & Thatcher, R. W. (2001). Frequency domain equivalence between potentials and currents using LORETA. *Int J Neurosci*, 107(3-4), 161-171.

Gordon, A. H., Lee, P. A., Dulcan, M. K., & Finegold, D. N. (1986). Behavioral problems, social competency, and self perception among girls with congenital adrenal hyperplasia. *Child Psychiatry Hum Dev*, 17(2), 129-138.

Gorman, J. M., Kent, J. M., Sullivan, G. M., & Coplan, J. D. (2000). Neuroanatomical hypothesis of panic disorder, revised. *Am J Psychiatry,* 157(4), 493-505.

Gotman, J., Grova, C., Bagshaw, A., Kobayashi, E., Aghakhani, Y., & Dubeau, F. (2005). Generalized epileptic discharges show thalamocortical activation and suspension of the default state of the brain. *Proc Natl Acad Sci U S A*, 102(42), 15236-15240.

Grady, C. L., Protzner, A. B., Kovacevic, N., Strother, S. C., Afshin-Pour, B., Wojtowicz, M., et al. (2009). A Multivariate Analysis of Age-Related Differences in Default Mode and Task-Positive Networks across Multiple Cognitive Domains. *Cereb Cortex.* 20:1432-1447

Grasby, P. M., Frith, C. D., Friston, K. J., Bench, C., Frackowiak, R. S., & Dolan, R. J. (1993). Functional mapping of brain areas implicated in auditory--verbal memory function. *Brain*, 116 (Pt 1), 1-20.

Greenblatt, D. J., Gan, L., Harmatz, J. S., & Shader, R. I. (2005). Pharmocokinetics and pharmacodynamics of single-dose triazolam: electroencephalography compared with the Digit-Symbol Substitution Test. *Br J Clin Pharmacol*, 60(3), 244-248.

Greicius, M. D., Krasnow, B., Reiss, A. L., & Menon, V. (2003). Functional connectivity in the resting brain: a network analysis of the default mode hypothesis. *Proc Natl Acad Sci U S A*, 100(1), 253-258.

Greicius, M. D., Srivastava, G., Reiss, A. L., & Menon, V. (2004). Default-mode network activity distinguishes Alzheimer's disease from healthy aging: evidence from functional MRI. *Proc Natl Acad Sci U S A,* 101(13), 4637-4642.

Griffin, L. D. (1994). The intrinsic geometry of the cerebral cortex. *J Theor Biol*, 166(3), 261-273.

Grillon, C. (2007). Models and mechanisms of anxiety: evidence from startle studies. *Psychopharmacology (Berl).* 199:421-437

Gruber, W. R., Klimesch, W., Sauseng, P., & Doppelmayr, M. (2005). Alpha phase synchronization predicts P1 and N1 latency and amplitude size. *Cereb Cortex*, 15(4), 371-377.

Guevara, M. A., Lorenzo, I., Arce, C., Ramos, J., & Corsi-Cabrera, M. (1995). Inter- and intrahemispheric EEG correlation during sleep and wakefulness. *Sleep*, 18(4), 257-265.

Gunnar, M. R. (1998). Quality of early care and buffering of neuroendocrine stress reactions: potential effects on the developing human brain. *Prev Med*, 27(2), 208-211.

Gusnard, D. A. (2005). Being a self: considerations from functional imaging. *Conscious Cogn*, 14(4), 679-697.

Gusnard, D. A., Akbudak, E., Shulman, G. L., & Raichle, M. E. (2001). Medial prefrontal cortex and self-referential mental activity: relation to a default mode of brain function. *Proc Natl Acad Sci U S A*, 98(7), 4259-4264.

Gusnard, D. A., Ollinger, J. M., Shulman, G. L., Cloninger, C. R., Price, J. L., Van Essen, D. C., et al. (2003). Persistence and brain circuitry. *Proc Natl Acad Sci U S A*, 100(6), 3479-3484.

Hale, J. R., Brookes, M. J., Hall, E. L., Zumer, J. M., Stevenson, C. M., Francis, S. T., et al. (2010). Comparison of functional connectivity in default mode and sensorimotor networks at 3 and 7T. *MAGMA*.23:339-349

Hamalainen, M. S., & Ilmoniemi, R. J. (1994). Interpreting magnetic fields of the brain: minimum norm estimates. *Med Biol Eng Comput*, 32(1), 35-42.

Hämäläinen, M. S. a. I., R.J. (1984). *Interpreting measured magnetic fields of the brain: estimates of current distributions*. Tech Rep. TKK-F-A559. Helsinki University of Technology.

Hammen, C. (2003). Interpersonal stress and depression in women. *J Affect Disord*, 74(1), 49-57.

Hanakawa, T., Honda, M., Sawamoto, N., Okada, T., Yonekura, Y., Fukuyama, H., et al. (2002). The role of rostral Brodmann area 6 in mental-operation tasks: an integrative neuroimaging approach. *Cereb Cortex*, 12(11), 1157-1170.

Hanaway, J., Woolsey, W.A., Gado, M.H., Melville, R.P., Jr. (1998). *The Brain Atlas: A Visual Guide to the Human Central Nervous System*. Bethesda: Fitzgerald Science Press.

Harmony, T., Fernandez, T., Silva, J., Bernal, J., Diaz-Comas, L., Reyes, A., et al. (1996). EEG delta activity: an indicator of attention to internal processing during performance of mental tasks. *Int J Psychophysiol,* 24(1-2), 161-171.

Harmony, T., Fernandez, T., Silva, J., Bosch, J., Valdes, P., Fernandez-Bouzas, A., et al. (1999). Do specific EEG frequencies indicate different processes during mental calculation? *Neurosci Lett*, 266(1), 25-28.

Haxby, J. V., Gobbini, M. I., Furey, M. L., Ishai, A., Schouten, J. L., & Pietrini, P. (2001). Distributed and overlapping representations of faces and objects in ventral temporal cortex. *Science*, 293(5539), 2425-2430.

Hazlett, E. A., Buchsbaum, M. S., Zhang, J., Newmark, R. E., Glanton, C. F., Zelmanova, Y., et al. (2008). Frontal-striatal-thalamic mediodorsal nucleus dysfunction in schizophrenia-spectrum patients during sensorimotor gating. *Neuroimage*, 42(3), 1164-1177.

Haznedar, M. M., Buchsbaum, M. S., Luu, C., Hazlett, E. A., Siegel, B. V., Jr., Lohr, J., et al. (1997). Decreased anterior cingulate gyrus metabolic rate in schizophrenia. *Am J Psychiatry*, 154(5), 682-684.

Hejmadi, A., Davidson, R. J., & Rozin, P. (2000). Exploring Hindu Indian emotion expressions: evidence for accurate recognition by Americans and Indians. *Psychol Sci*, 11(3), 183-187.

Helmeke, C., Ovtscharoff, W., Jr., Poeggel, G., & Braun, K. (2001). Juvenile emotional experience alters synaptic inputs on pyramidal neurons in the anterior cingulate cortex. *Cereb Cortex*, 11(8), 717-727.

Helmeke, C., Poeggel, G., & Braun, K. (2001). Differential emotional experience induces elevated spine densities on basal dendrites of pyramidal neurons in the anterior cingulate cortex of Octodon degus. *Neuroscience, 104(4), 927-931.*

Henriques, J. B., & Davidson, R. J. (1991). Left frontal hypoactivation in depression. *J Abnorm Psychol*, 100(4), 535-545.

Herman, J. P., & Cullinan, W. E. (1997). Neurocircuitry of stress: central control of the hypothalamo-pituitary-adrenocortical axis. *Trends Neurosci, 20(2), 78-84.*

Herman, J. P., Figueiredo, H., Mueller, N. K., Ulrich-Lai, Y., Ostrander, M. M., Choi, D. C., et al. (2003). Central mechanisms of stress integration: hierarchical circuitry controlling hypothalamo-pituitary-adrenocortical responsiveness. *Front Neuroendocrinol*, 24(3), 151-180.

Herman, J. P., Flak, J., & Jankord, R. (2008). Chronic stress plasticity in the hypothalamic paraventricular nucleus. *Prog Brain Res*, 170, 353-364.

Herman, J. P., Renda, A., & Bodie, B. (2003). Norepinephrine-gamma-aminobutyric acid (GABA) interaction in limbic stress circuits: effects of reboxetine on GABAergic neurons. *Biol Psychiatry, 53(2), 166-174.*

Hermann, J., Gulati, R., Napoli, C., Woodrum, J. E., Lerman, L. O., Rodriguez-Porcel, M., et al. (2003). Oxidative stress-related increase in ubiquitination in early coronary atherogenesis. *FASEB J*, 17(12), 1730-1732.

Hernandez-Reif, M., Field, T., Diego, M., Vera, Y., & Pickens, J. (2006). Happy faces are habituated more slowly by infants of depressed mothers. *Infant Behav Dev*, 29(1), 131-135.

Herning, R. I., Glover, B. J., Koeppl, B., Phillips, R. L., & London, E. D. (1994). Cocaine-induced increases in EEG alpha and beta activity: evidence for reduced cortical processing. *Neuropsychopharmacology*, 11(1), 1-9.

Herning, R. I., Jones, R. T., Hooker, W. D., Mendelson, J., & Blackwell, L. (1985). Cocaine increases EEG beta: a replication and extension of Hans Berger's historic experiments. *Electroencephalogr Clin Neurophysiol*, 60(6), 470-477.

Herning, R. I., & King, D. E. (1996). EEG and evoked potentials alterations in cocaine-dependent individuals. *NIDA Res Monogr*, 163, 203-223.

Hesslinger, B., Tebartz van Elst, L., Thiel, T., Haegele, K., Hennig, J., & Ebert, D. (2002). Frontoorbital volume reductions in adult patients with attention deficit hyperactivity disorder. *Neurosci Lett*, 328(3), 319-321.

Holloway, M. (2003). The mutable brain. *Sci Am*, 289(3), 78-85.

Holmes, M. D., Brown, M., & Tucker, D. M. (2004). Are "generalized" seizures truly generalized? Evidence of localized mesial frontal and frontopolar discharges in absence. *Epilepsia*, 45(12), 1568-1579.

Holsboer, F. (2001). Stress, hypercortisolism and corticosteroid receptors in depression: implications for therapy. *J Affect Disord*, 62(1-2), 77-91.

Horner, B. R., & Scheibe, K. E. (1997). Prevalence and implications of attention-deficit hyperactivity disorder among adolescents in treatment for substance abuse. *J Am Acad Child Adolesc Psychiatry*, 36(1), 30-36.

Hughes, J. R. (1995). The EEG in psychiatry: an outline with summarized points and references. *Clin Electroencephalogr*, 26(2), 92-101.

Hughes, J. R. (1996). A review of the usefulness of the standard EEG in psychiatry. *Clin Electroencephalogr,* 27(1), 35-39.

Hughes, J. R., & John, E. R. (1999). Conventional and quantitative electroencephalography in psychiatry. *J Neuropsychiatry Clin Neurosci,* 11(2), 190-208.

Hull, E. M., Du, J., Lorrain, D. S., & Matuszewich, L. (1995). Extracellular dopamine in the medial preoptic area: implications for sexual motivation and hormonal control of copulation. *J Neurosci*, 15(11), 7465-7471.

Hung, J. H., Whitfield, T. W., Yang, T. H., Hu, Z., Weng, Z., & DeLisi, C. (2010). Identification of functional modules that correlate with phenotypic difference: the influence of network topology. *Genome Biol*, 11(2), R23.

Iannetti, G. D., Porro, C. A., Pantano, P., Romanelli, P. L., Galeotti, F., & Cruccu, G. (2003). Representation of different trigeminal divisions within the primary and secondary human somatosensory cortex. *Neuroimage*, 19(3), 906-912.

Ikemoto, S. (2007). Dopamine reward circuitry: two projection systems from the ventral midbrain to the nucleus accumbens-olfactory tubercle complex. *Brain Res Rev,* 56(1), 27-78.

Isa, T., & Sasaki, S. (2002). Brainstem control of head movements during orienting; organization of the premotor circuits. *Prog Neurobiol*, 66(4), 205-241.

Isaacman, D. J., Poirier, M. P., Loiselle, J. M., & Schutzman, S. (2002). Closed head injury in children. *Pediatr Emerg Care*, 18(1), 48-52.

Isotani, T., Tanaka, H., Lehmann, D., Pascual-Marqui, R. D., Kochi, K., Saito, N., et al. (2001). Source localization of EEG activity during hypnotically induced anxiety and relaxation. *Int J Psychophysiol*, 41(2), 143-153.

Itokawa, M., & Yoshikawa, T. (2007). Molecular biology of depressive disorders. *Nippon Rinsho*, 65(9), 1599-1606.

Izard, C. E., Libero, D. Z., Putnam, P., & Haynes, O. M. (1993). Stability of emotion experiences and their relations to traits of personality. *J Pers Soc Psychol*, 64(5), 847-860.

Jacobus, J., McQueeny, T., Bava, S., Schweinsburg, B. C., Frank, L. R., Yang, T. T., et al. (2009). White matter integrity in adolescents with histories of marijuana use and binge drinking. *Neurotoxicol Teratol*, 31(6), 349-355.

Jahanshahi, M., Dirnberger, G., Fuller, R., & Frith, C. D. (2000). The role of the dorsolateral prefrontal cortex in random number generation: a study with positron emission tomography. *Neuroimage*, 12(6), 713-725.

Jankord, R., & Herman, J. P. (2008). Limbic regulation of hypothalamo-pituitary-adrenocortical function during acute and chronic stress. *Ann N Y Acad Sci*, 1148, 64-73.

Jansen, B. H., Hegde, A., & Boutros, N. N. (2004). Contribution of different EEG frequencies to auditory evoked potential abnormalities in schizophrenia. *Clin Neurophysiol,* 115(3), 523-533.

Jasper, H. (1958). Progress and problems in brain research. *J Mt Sinai Hosp N Y*, 25(3), 244-253.

Jausovec, N., & Jausovec, K. (2001). Differences in EEG current density related to intelligence. *Brain Res Cogn Brain Res*, 12(1), 55-60.

Jensen, O., & Tesche, C. D. (2002). Frontal theta activity in humans increases with memory load in a working memory task. *Eur J Neurosci*, 15(8), 1395-1399.

Jeong, J. (2004). EEG dynamics in patients with Alzheimer's disease. *Clin Neurophysiol,* 115(7), 1490-1505.

Jerlhag, E., Egecioglu, E., Dickson, S. L., Andersson, M., Svensson, L., & Engel, J. A. (2006). Ghrelin stimulates locomotor activity and accumbal dopamine-overflow via central cholinergic systems in mice: implications for its involvement in brain reward. *Addict Biol*, 11(1), 45-54.

Joels, M., Krugers, H., & Karst, H. (2007). Stress-induced changes in hippocampal function. *Prog Brain Res*, 167, 3-15.

Jog, M. S., Kubota, Y., Connolly, C. I., Hillegaart, V., & Graybiel, A. M. (1999). Building neural representations of habits. *Science*, 286(5445), 1745-1749.

John, E. R. (1989). The role of quantitative EEG topographic mapping or 'neurometrics' in the diagnosis of psychiatric and neurological disorders: the pros. *Electroencephalogr Clin Neurophysiol*, 73(1), 2-4.

John, E. R., Prichep, L. S., Fridman, J., & Easton, P. (1988). Neurometrics: computer-assisted differential diagnosis of brain dysfunctions. Science, 239(4836), 162-169.

Johnson, D. (1994). Stress, depression, substance abuse, and racism. *Am Indian Alsk Native Ment Health Res*, 6(1), 29-33.

Johnson, T. L., Wright, S. C., & Segall, A. (1979). Filtering of muscle artifact from the electroencephalogram. *IEEE Trans Biomed Eng*, 26(10), 556-563.

Jones, S. R., Pinto, D. J., Kaper, T. J., & Kopell, N. (2000). Alpha-frequency rhythms desynchronize over long cortical distances: a modeling study. *J Comput Neurosci,* 9(3), 271-291.

Jones, S. S. (2009). The development of imitation in infancy. *Philos Trans R Soc Lond B Biol Sci,* 364(1528), 2325-2335.

Joyce, C. A., Gorodnitsky, I. F., & Kutas, M. (2004). Automatic removal of eye movement and blink artifacts from EEG data using blind component separation. *Psychophysiology*, 41(2), 313-325.

Just, M. A., Cherkassky, V. L., Keller, T. A., Kana, R. K., & Minshew, N. J. (2007). Functional and anatomical cortical underconnectivity in autism: evidence from an FMRI study of an executive function task and corpus callosum morphometry. *Cereb Cortex*, 17(4), 951-961.

Kackar, R. N., Harville, D.A. (1984). Approximations for Standard Errors of Estimators of Fixed and Random Effects in Mixed Linear Models. *Journal of the American Statistical Association*, 79(388), 853-862.

Kaiser, D. A. (2007). What Is Quantitative EEG? *Journal of Neurotherapy: Investigations in Neuromodulation, Neurofeedback and Applied Neuroscience*, 10(4), 37 - 52.

Kalin, N. H., Larson, C., Shelton, S. E., & Davidson, R. J. (1998). Asymmetric frontal brain activity, cortisol, and behavior associated with fearful temperament in rhesus monkeys. *Behav Neurosci*, 112(2), 286-292.

Kalin, N. H., Shelton, S. E., & Barksdale, C. M. (1987). Separation distress in infant rhesus monkeys: effects of diazepam and Ro 15-1788. *Brain Res*, 408(1-2), 192-198.

Kalin, N. H., Shelton, S. E., & Davidson, R. J. (2000). Cerebrospinal fluid corticotropin-releasing hormone levels are elevated in monkeys with patterns of brain activity associated with fearful temperament. *Biol Psychiatry*, 47(7), 579-585.

Kanai, R., Lloyd, H., Bueti, D., & Walsh, V. (2011). Modality-independent role of the primary auditory cortex in time estimation. *Exp Brain Res.* 209:465-471

Kaneda, M., & Osaka, N. (2008). Role of anterior cingulate cortex during semantic coding in verbal working memory. *Neurosci Lett,* 436(1), 57-61.

Kelley, W. M., Macrae, C. N., Wyland, C. L., Caglar, S., Inati, S., & Heatherton, T. F. (2002). Finding the self? An event-related fMRI study. *J Cogn Neurosci*, 14(5), 785-794.

Kelley, W. M., Miezin, F. M., McDermott, K. B., Buckner, R. L., Raichle, M. E., Cohen, N. J., et al. (1998). Hemispheric specialization in human dorsal frontal cortex and medial temporal lobe for verbal and nonverbal memory encoding. *Neuron*, 20(5), 927-936.

Kennerley, S. W., Walton, M. E., Behrens, T. E., Buckley, M. J., & Rushworth, M. F. (2006). Optimal decision making and the anterior cingulate cortex. *Nat Neurosci*, 9(7), 940-947.

Kenny, P. J., Chartoff, E., Roberto, M., Carlezon, W. A., Jr., & Markou, A. (2009). NMDA receptors regulate nicotine-enhanced brain reward function and intravenous nicotine self-administration: role of the ventral tegmental area and central nucleus of the amygdala. *Neuropsychopharmacology*, 34(2), 266-281.

Kensinger, E. A., & Schacter, D. L. (2005). Emotional content and reality-monitoring ability: fMRI evidence for the influences of encoding processes. *Neuropsychologia*, 43(10), 1429-1443.

Kern, S., Oakes, T. R., Stone, C. K., McAuliff, E. M., Kirschbaum, C., & Davidson, R. J. (2008). Glucose metabolic changes in the prefrontal cortex are associated with HPA axis response to a psychosocial stressor. *Psychoneuroendocrinology*, 33(4), 517-529.

Kim, E. Y., Kim, D. H., Chang, J. H., Yoo, E., Lee, J. W., & Park, H. J. (2009). Triple-layer appearance of Brodmann area 4 at thin-section double inversion-recovery MR imaging. *Radiology*, 250(2), 515-522.

Kim, S. H., & Hamann, S. (2007). Neural correlates of positive and negative emotion regulation. *J Cogn Neurosci,* 19(5), 776-798.

Kim, Y. Y., Roh, A. Y., Namgoong, Y., Jo, H. J., Lee, J. M., & Kwon, J. S. (2009). Cortical network dynamics during source memory retrieval: current density imaging with individual MRI. *Hum Brain Mapp*, 30(1), 78-91.

Kircher, T. T., & Leube, D. T. (2003). Self-consciousness, self-agency, and schizophrenia. *Conscious Cogn*, 12(4), 656-669.

Kircher, T. T., Seiferth, N. Y., Plewnia, C., Baar, S., & Schwabe, R. (2007). Self-face recognition in schizophrenia. *Schizophr Res,* 94(1-3), 264-272.

Kirimoto, H., Ogata, K., Onishi, H., Oyama, M., Goto, Y., & Tobimatsu, S. (2010). Transcranial direct current stimulation over the motor association cortex induces plastic changes in ipsilateral primary motor and somatosensory cortices. *Clin Neurophysiol*. 122-777-783

Kirsch, P., Schienle, A., Stark, R., Sammer, G., Blecker, C., Walter, B., et al. (2003). Anticipation of reward in a nonaversive differential conditioning paradigm and the brain reward system: an event-related fMRI study. *Neuroimage*, 20(2), 1086-1095.

Kirwan, C. B., Bayley, P. J., Galvan, V. V., & Squire, L. R. (2008). Detailed recollection of remote autobiographical memory after damage to the medial temporal lobe. *Proc Natl Acad Sci U S A*.

Klimesch, W. (1996). Memory processes, brain oscillations and EEG synchronization. *Int J Psychophysiol*, 24(1-2), 61-100.

Klimesch, W. (1997). EEG-alpha rhythms and memory processes. *Int J Psychophysiol,* 26(1-3), 319-340.

Klimesch, W. (1999). EEG alpha and theta oscillations reflect cognitive and memory performance: a review and analysis. *Brain Res Brain Res Rev, 29*(2-3), 169-195.

Klimesch, W. (1999). EEG alpha and theta oscillations reflect cognitive and memory performance: A review and analysis. *Brain Research Reviews, 29*(2), 169-195.

Klimesch, W. (2000). *Theta frequency, synchronization and episodic memory performance. In R. Miller (Ed.), Time and the Brain* (pp. 225-339). Australia: Harwood Academic Publishers.

Klimesch, W., Doppelmayr, M., Pachinger, T., & Ripper, B. (1997). Brain oscillations and human memory: EEG correlates in the upper alpha and theta band. *Neurosci Lett, 238*(1-2), 9-12.

Klimesch, W., Doppelmayr, M., Russegger, H., & Pachinger, T. (1996). Theta band power in the human scalp EEG and the encoding of new information. *Neuroreport, 7*(7), 1235-1240.

Klimesch, W., Doppelmayr, M., Russegger, H., Pachinger, T., & Schwaiger, J. (1998). Induced alpha band power changes in the human EEG and attention. *Neurosci Lett, 244*(2), 73-76.

Klimesch, W., Doppelmayr, M., Schimke, H., & Ripper, B. (1997). Theta synchronization and alpha desynchronization in a memory task. *Psychophysiology, 34*(2), 169-176.

Klimesch, W., Doppelmayr, M., Schwaiger, J., Auinger, P., & Winkler, T. (1999). 'Paradoxical' alpha synchronization in a memory task. *Cognitive Brain Research, 7*(4), 493-501.

Klimesch, W., Doppelmayr, M., Stadler, M., Pollhuber, P., Sauseng, P., & Rohm, D. (2001). Episodic retrieval is reflected by a process specific increase in human electroencephalographic theta activity. *Neuroscience Letters, 302*, 49-52.

Klimesch, W., Hanslmayr, S., Sauseng, P., Gruber, W., Brozinsky, C. J., Kroll, N. E., et al. (2006). Oscillatory EEG correlates of episodic trace decay. *Cereb Cortex, 16*(2), 280-290.

Klimesch, W., Sauseng, P., & Gerloff, C. (2003). Enhancing cognitive performance with repetitive transcranial magnetic stimulation at human individual alpha frequency. *European Journal of Neuroscience, 17*, 1129-1133.

Klimesch, W., Schack, B., & Sauseng, P. (2005). The functional significance of theta and upper alpha oscillations. *Exp Psychol, 52*(2), 99-108.

Klimesch, W., Schimke, H., & Schwaiger, J. (1994). Episodic and semantic memory: an analysis in the EEG theta and alpha band. *Electroencephalogr Clin Neurophysiol, 91*(6), 428-441.

Knyazev, G. G., Savostyanov, A. N., & Levin, E. A. (2005). Uncertainty, anxiety, and brain oscillations. *Neurosci Lett, 387*(3), 121-125.

Kohler, S., Paus, T., Buckner, R. L., & Milner, B. (2004). Effects of left inferior prefrontal stimulation on episodic memory formation: a two-stage fMRI-rTMS study. *J Cogn Neurosci, 16*(2), 178-188.

Kolev, V., Demiralp, T., Yordanova, J., Ademoglu, A., & Isoglu-Alkac, U. (1997). Time-frequency analysis reveals multiple functional components during oddball P300. *Neuroreport,* 8(8), 2061-2065.

Komisaruk, B. R., & Whipple, B. (2005). Functional MRI of the brain during orgasm in women. *Annu Rev Sex Res,* 16, 62-86.

Konrad, K., Neufang, S., Hanisch, C., Fink, G. R., & Herpertz-Dahlmann, B. (2006). Dysfunctional attentional networks in children with attention deficit/hyperactivity disorder: evidence from an event-related functional magnetic resonance imaging study. *Biol Psychiatry,* 59(7), 643-651.

Kopell, N., Ermentrout, G. B., Whittington, M. A., & Traub, R. D. (2000). Gamma rhythms and beta rhythms have different synchronization properties. *Proc Natl Acad Sci U S A,* 97(4), 1867-1872.

Koskinen, M., & Vartiainen, N. (2009). Removal of imaging artifacts in EEG during simultaneous EEG/fMRI recording: reconstruction of a high-precision artifact template. *Neuroimage,* 46(1), 160-167.

Kotz, S. A., D'Ausilio, A., Raettig, T., Begliomini, C., Craighero, L., Fabbri-Destro, M., et al. (2010). Lexicality drives audio-motor transformations in Broca's area. *Brain Lang,* 112(1), 3-11.

Krause, B. J., Hautzel, H., Schmidt, D., Fluss, M. O., Poeppel, T. D., Muller, H. W., et al. (2006). Learning related interactions among neuronal systems involved in memory processes. *J Physiol Paris,* 99(4-6), 318-332.

Kurova, N. S., & Cheremushkin, E. A. (2007). Spectral EEG characteristics during increases in the complexity of the context of cognitive activity. *Neurosci Behav Physiol,* 37(4), 379-385.

Kurth, R., Villringer, K., Mackert, B. M., Schwiemann, J., Braun, J., Curio, G., et al. (1998). fMRI assessment of somatotopy in human Brodmann area 3b by electrical finger stimulation. *Neuroreport,* 9(2), 207-212.

Lacerda, A. L., Hardan, A. Y., Yorbik, O., Vemulapalli, M., Prasad, K. M., & Keshavan, M. S. (2007). Morphology of the orbitofrontal cortex in first-episode schizophrenia: relationship with negative symptomatology. *Prog Neuropsychopharmacol Biol Psychiatry,* 31(2), 510-516.

Lahiri, P., Rao, J.N.K. (1995). Robust Estimation of Mean Squared Error of Small Area Estimators. *Journal of the American Statistical Association,* 90(430), 758-766.

Lancaster, J. L., Woldorff, M. G., Parsons, L. M., Liotti, M., Freitas, C. S., Rainey, L., et al. (2000). Automated Talairach atlas labels for functional brain mapping. *Hum Brain Mapp,* 10(3), 120-131.

Lang, P. J. (1979). Presidential address, 1978. A bio-informational theory of emotional imagery. *Psychophysiology,* 16(6), 495-512.

Lang, P. J., Kozak, M. J., Miller, G. A., Levin, D. N., & McLean, A., Jr. (1980). Emotional imagery: conceptual structure and pattern of somato-visceral response. *Psychophysiology*, 17(2), 179-192.

Lansbergen, M. M., Arns, M., van Dongen-Boomsma, M., Spronk, D., & Buitelaar, J. K. (2010). The increase in theta/beta ratio on resting-state EEG in boys with attention-deficit/hyperactivity disorder is mediated by slow alpha peak frequency. P*rog Neuropsychopharmacol Biol Psychiatry*. 35:47-52

Laviolette, S. R., & van der Kooy, D. (2004). GABAA receptors signal bidirectional reward transmission from the ventral tegmental area to the tegmental pedunculopontine nucleus as a function of opiate state. *Eur J Neurosci,* 20(8), 2179-2187.

Lawrence, A. D., Evans, A. H., & Lees, A. J. (2003). Compulsive use of dopamine replacement therapy in Parkinson's disease: reward systems gone awry? *Lancet Neurol*, 2(10), 595-604.

Learmonth, A. E., Lamberth, R., & Rovee-Collier, C. (2005). The social context of imitation in infancy. *J Exp Child Psychol*, 91(4), 297-314.

LeDoux, J. (1998). Fear and the brain: where have we been, and where are we going? Biol Psychiatry, 44(12), 1229-1238.

LeDoux, J. E., Cicchetti, P., Xagoraris, A., & Romanski, L. M. (1990). The lateral amygdaloid nucleus: sensory interface of the amygdala in fear conditioning. *J Neurosci*, 10(4), 1062-1069.

LeDoux, J. E., Farb, C., & Ruggiero, D. A. (1990). Topographic organization of neurons in the acoustic thalamus that project to the amygdala. *J Neurosci*, 10(4), 1043-1054.

LeDoux, J. E., & Gorman, J. M. (2001). A call to action: overcoming anxiety through active coping. *Am J Psychiatry*, 158(12), 1953-1955.

Lehmann, D., Faber, P. L., Achermann, P., Jeanmonod, D., Gianotti, L. R., & Pizzagalli, D. (2001). Brain sources of EEG gamma frequency during volitionally meditation-induced, altered states of consciousness, and experience of the self. *Psychiatry Res*, 108(2), 111-121.

Lehmann, D., Faber, P. L., Galderisi, S., Herrmann, W. M., Kinoshita, T., Koukkou, M., et al. (2005). EEG microstate duration and syntax in acute, medication-naive, first-episode schizophrenia: a multi-center study. *Psychiatry Res,* 138(2), 141-156.

Lehmann, D., Faber, P. L., Gianotti, L. R., Kochi, K., & Pascual-Marqui, R. D. (2006). Coherence and phase locking in the scalp EEG and between LORETA model sources, and microstates as putative mechanisms of brain temporo-spatial functional organization. J *Physiol Paris,* 99(1), 29-36.

Lehmann, D., Henggeler, B., Koukkou, M., & Michel, C. M. (1993). Source localization of brain electric field frequency bands during conscious, spontaneous, visual imagery and abstract thought. *Brain Res Cogn Brain Res*, 1(4), 203-210.

Lehmann, D., Michel, C. M., Pal, I., & Pascual-Marqui, R. D. (1994). Event-related potential maps depend on prestimulus brain electric microstate map. *Int J Neurosci*, 74(1-4), 239-248.

Leiner, H. C., Leiner, A. L., & Dow, R. S. (1989). Reappraising the cerebellum: what does the hindbrain contribute to the forebrain? *Behav Neurosci*, 103(5), 998-1008.

Leung, L. W., & Borst, J. G. (1987). Electrical activity of the cingulate cortex. I. Generating mechanisms and relations to behavior. *Brain Res*, 407(1), 68-80.

Levesque, J., Beauregard, M., & Mensour, B. (2006). Effect of neurofeedback training on the neural substrates of selective attention in children with attention-deficit/hyperactivity disorder: a functional magnetic resonance imaging study. *Neurosci Lett*, 394(3), 216-221.

Levesque, J., Eugene, F., Joanette, Y., Paquette, V., Mensour, B., Beaudoin, G., et al. (2003). Neural circuitry underlying voluntary suppression of sadness. *Biol Psychiatry*, 53(6), 502-510.

Levin, F. R., & Kleber, H. D. (1995). Attention-deficit hyperactivity disorder and substance abuse: relationships and implications for treatment. *Harv Rev Psychiatry*, 2(5), 246-258.

Levitin, D. J., & Menon, V. (2003). Musical structure is processed in "language" areas of the brain: a possible role for Brodmann Area 47 in temporal coherence. Neuroimage, 20(4), 2142-2152.

Liberzon, I., Phan, K. L., Decker, L. R., & Taylor, S. F. (2003). Extended amygdala and emotional salience: a PET activation study of positive and negative affect. N*europsychopharmacology*, 28(4), 726-733.

Liddell, B. J., Brown, K. J., Kemp, A. H., Barton, M. J., Das, P., Peduto, A., et al. (2005). A direct brainstem-amygdala-cortical 'alarm' system for subliminal signals of fear. *Neuroimage*, 24(1), 235-243.

Liddle, P. F. (1992). PET scanning and schizophrenia--what progress? *Psychol Med*, 22(3), 557-560.

Liddle, P. F., Friston, K. J., Frith, C. D., & Frackowiak, R. S. (1992). Cerebral blood flow and mental processes in schizophrenia. *J R Soc Med*, 85(4), 224-227.

Liegeois, F., Connelly, A., Cross, J. H., Boyd, S. G., Gadian, D. G., Vargha-Khadem, F., et al. (2004). Language reorganization in children with early-onset lesions of the left hemisphere: an fMRI study. *Brain*, 127(Pt 6), 1229-1236.

Liotti, M., Mayberg, H. S., McGinnis, S., Brannan, S. L., & Jerabek, P. (2002). Unmasking disease-specific cerebral blood flow abnormalities: mood challenge in patients with remitted unipolar depression. *Am J Psychiatry*, 159(11), 1830-1840.

Liverant, G. I., Brown, T. A., Barlow, D. H., & Roemer, L. (2008). Emotion regulation in unipolar depression: the effects of acceptance and suppression of subjective emotional experience on the intensity and duration of sadness and negative affect. *Behav Res Ther*, 46(11), 1201-1209.

Ljungberg, T., Apicella, P., & Schultz, W. (1992). Responses of monkey dopamine neurons during learning of behavioral reactions. *J Neurophysiol*, 67(1), 145-163.

Lodge, D. J., & Grace, A. A. (2006). The laterodorsal tegmentum is essential for burst firing of ventral tegmental area dopamine neurons. *Proc Natl Acad Sci U S A*, 103(13), 5167-5172.

Logothetis, N. K., Pauls, J., Augath, M., Trinath, T., & Oeltermann, A. (2001). Neurophysiological investigation of the basis of the fMRI signal. *Nature,* 412(6843), 150-157.

Logothetis, N. K., & Wandell, B. A. (2004). Interpreting the BOLD signal. *Annu Rev Physiol,* 66, 735-769.

Lopes da Silva, F. (2004). Functional localization of brain sources using EEG and/or MEG data: volume conductor and source models. *Magnetic Resonance Imaging*, 22(10), 1533-1538.

Lubar, J. F. (1997). Neocortical dynamics: implications for understanding the role of neurofeedback and related techniques for the enhancement of attention. *Appl Psychophysiol Biofeedback*, 22(2), 111-126.

Lubar, J. F., Congedo, M., & Askew, J. H. (2003). Low-resolution electromagnetic tomography (LORETA) of cerebral activity in chronic depressive disorder. *Int J Psychophysiol*, 49(3), 175-185.

Lubin, A., Nute, C., Naitoh, P., & Martin, W. B. (1973). EEG delta activity during human sleep as a damped ultradian rhythm. *Psychophysiology*, 10(1), 27-35.

Lukas, S. E., Mendelson, J. H., Amass, L., & Benedikt, R. (1989). Behavioral and EEG studies of acute cocaine administration: comparisons with morphine, amphetamine, pentobarbital, nicotine, ethanol and marijuana. *NIDA Res Monogr,* 95, 146-151.

Luria, A. R. (1966). *Higher Cortical Functions in Man* (Second ed.). New York: Basic Books Inc.

Lustig, C., Snyder, A. Z., Bhakta, M., O'Brien, K. C., McAvoy, M., Raichle, M. E., et al. (2003). Functional deactivations: change with age and dementia of the Alzheimer type. *Proc Natl Acad Sci U S A,* 100(24), 14504-14509.

Lutkenhoner, B. (2011). Auditory signal detection appears to depend on temporal integration of subthreshold activity in auditory cortex. *Brain Res*. 1385:206-246

Lutz, A., Greischar, L. L., Perlman, D., & Davidson, R. J. (2009). BOLD signal in insula is differentially related to cardiac function during compassion meditation in experts vs. novices. *Neuroimage*. 47:1038-1046

Luu, P., & Posner, M. I. (2003). Anterior cingulate cortex regulation of sympathetic activity. *Brain*, 126(Pt 10), 2119-2120.

MacDonald, A. W., 3rd, Cohen, J. D., Stenger, V. A., & Carter, C. S. (2000). Dissociating the role of the dorsolateral prefrontal and anterior cingulate cortex in cognitive control. *Science*, 288(5472), 1835-1838.

Machulda, M. M., Ward, H. A., Borowski, B., Gunter, J. L., Cha, R. H., O'Brien, P. C., et al. (2003). Comparison of memory fMRI response among normal, MCI, and Alzheimer's patients. *Neurology, 61*(4), 500-506.

Maddock, R. J. (1999). The retrosplenial cortex and emotion: new insights from functional neuroimaging of the human brain. *Trends Neurosci, 22*(7), 310-316.

Maletic, V., Robinson, M., Oakes, T., Iyengar, S., Ball, S. G., & Russell, J. (2007). Neurobiology of depression: an integrated view of key findings. *Int J Clin Pract, 61*(12), 2030-2040.

Mannuzza, S., Fyer, A. J., Martin, L. Y., Gallops, M. S., Endicott, J., Gorman, J., et al. (1989). Reliability of anxiety assessment. I. *Diagnostic agreement. Arch Gen Psychiatry, 46*(12), 1093-1101.

Mannuzza, S., Klein, R. G., Konig, P. H., & Giampino, T. L. (1989). Hyperactive boys almost grown up. IV. Criminality and its relationship to psychiatric status. *Arch Gen Psychiatry, 46*(12), 1073-1079.

Marcus, S. M., Young, E. A., Kerber, K. B., Kornstein, S., Farabaugh, A. H., Mitchell, J., et al. (2005). Gender differences in depression: findings from the STAR*D study. *J Affect Disord, 87*(2-3), 141-150.

Matousek, M., Brunovsky, M., Edman, A., & Wallin, A. (2001). EEG abnormalities in dementia reflect the parietal lobe syndrome. *Clin Neurophysiol, 112*(6), 1001-1005.

Mayberg, H. S., Silva, J. A., Brannan, S. K., Tekell, J. L., Mahurin, R. K., McGinnis, S., et al. (2002). The functional neuroanatomy of the placebo effect. *Am J Psychiatry, 159*(5), 728-737.

Mayes, L. C. (1999). Addressing mental health needs of infants and young children. *Child Adolesc Psychiatr Clin N Am, 8*(2), 209-224.

Mazerolle, E. L., Beyea, S. D., Gawryluk, J. R., Brewer, K. D., Bowen, C. V., & D'Arcy, R. C. (2010). Confirming white matter fMRI activation in the corpus callosum: co-localization with DTI tractography. *Neuroimage, 50*(2), 616-621.

McAlonan, G. M., Cheung, V., Cheung, C., Chua, S. E., Murphy, D. G., Suckling, J., et al. (2007). Mapping brain structure in attention deficit-hyperactivity disorder: a voxel-based MRI study of regional grey and white matter volume. *Psychiatry Res, 154*(2), 171-180.

McCaslin, A. F., Chen, B. R., Radosevich, A. J., Cauli, B., & Hillman, E. M. (2010). In vivo 3D morphology of astrocyte-vasculature interactions in the somatosensory cortex: implications for neurovascular coupling. *J Cereb Blood Flow Metab*.31:795-806

McCrone, J. (2002). The first word. *Lancet Neurol, 1*(1), 72.

McEwen, B. S. (1998). Stress, adaptation, and disease. Allostasis and allostatic load. *Ann N Y Acad Sci, 840*, 33-44.

McEwen, B. S. (2000a). The neurobiology of stress: from serendipity to clinical relevance. *Brain Res, 886*(1-2), 172-189.

McEwen, B. S. (2000b). Protective and damaging effects of stress mediators: central role of the brain. *Prog Brain Res*, 122, 25-34.

Medina, K. L., Nagel, B. J., Park, A., McQueeny, T., & Tapert, S. F. (2007). Depressive symptoms in adolescents: associations with white matter volume and marijuana use. *J Child Psychol Psychiatry*, 48(6), 592-600.

Meltzoff, A. N. (1990). Towards a developmental cognitive science. The implications of cross-modal matching and imitation for the development of representation and memory in infancy. *Ann N Y Acad Sci*, 608, 1-31; discussion 31-37.

Mesulam, M. M. (1990). Large-scale neurocognitive networks and distributed processing for attention, language, and memory. *Ann Neurol,* 28(5), 597-613.

Middleton, F. A., & Strick, P. L. (1994). Anatomical evidence for cerebellar and basal ganglia involvement in higher cognitive function. *Science*, 266(5184), 458-461.

Mientus, S., Gallinat, J., Wuebben, Y., Pascual-Marqui, R. D., Mulert, C., Frick, K., et al. (2002). Cortical hypoactivation during resting EEG in schizophrenics but not in depressives and schizotypal subjects as revealed by low resolution electromagnetic tomography (LORETA). *Psychiatry Res*, 116(1-2), 95-111.

Miguel-Hidalgo, J. J., & Rajkowska, G. (2003). Comparison of prefrontal cell pathology between depression and alcohol dependence. *J Psychiatr Res*, 37(5), 411-420.

Milad, M. R., & Rauch, S. L. (2007). The role of the orbitofrontal cortex in anxiety disorders. *Ann N Y Acad Sci,* 1121, 546-561.

Miltner, W., Braun, C., Johnson, R., Jr., Simpson, G. V., & Ruchkin, D. S. (1994). A test of brain electrical source analysis (BESA): a simulation study. *Electroencephalogr Clin Neurophysiol*, 91(4), 295-310.

Mitchell, J. B., & Gratton, A. (1994). Involvement of mesolimbic dopamine neurons in sexual behaviors: implications for the neurobiology of motivation. *Rev Neurosci*, 5(4), 317-329.

Mobbs, D., Greicius, M. D., Abdel-Azim, E., Menon, V., & Reiss, A. L. (2003). Humor modulates the mesolimbic reward centers. *Neuron*, 40(5), 1041-1048.

Monastra, V. J. (2005). Electroencephalographic biofeedback (neurotherapy) as a treatment for attention deficit hyperactivity disorder: rationale and empirical foundation. *Child Adolesc Psychiatr Clin N Am,* 14(1), 55-82, vi.

Monastra, V. J. (2008). Quantitative electroencephalography and attention-deficit/hyperactivity disorder: implications for clinical practice. *Curr Psychiatry Rep*, 10(5), 432-438.

Monastra, V. J., Lubar, J. F., & Linden, M. (2001). The development of a quantitative electroencephalographic scanning process for attention deficit-hyperactivity disorder: reliability and validity studies. *Neuropsychology*, 15(1), 136-144.

Monastra, V. J., Lubar, J. F., Linden, M., VanDeusen, P., Green, G., Wing, W., et al. (1999). Assessing attention deficit hyperactivity disorder via quantitative electroencephalography: an initial validation study. *Neuropsychology*, 13(3), 424-433.

Monastra, V. J., Lynn, S., Linden, M., Lubar, J. F., Gruzelier, J., & LaVaque, T. J. (2005). Electroencephalographic biofeedback in the treatment of attention-deficit/hyperactivity disorder. *Appl Psychophysiol Biofeedback,* 30(2), 95-114.

Monastra, V. J., Monastra, D. M., & George, S. (2002). The effects of stimulant therapy, EEG biofeedback, and parenting style on the primary symptoms of attention-deficit/hyperactivity disorder. *Appl Psychophysiol Biofeedback*, 27(4), 231-249.

Money, J. (1973). Turner's syndrome and parietal lobe functions. *Cortex*, 9(4), 387-393.

Moran, J. M., Wig, G. S., Adams, R. B., Jr., Janata, P., & Kelley, W. M. (2004). Neural correlates of humor detection and appreciation. *Neuroimage*, 21(3), 1055-1060.

Moriguchi, Y., Ohnishi, T., Lane, R. D., Maeda, M., Mori, T., Nemoto, K., et al. (2006). Impaired self-awareness and theory of mind: an fMRI study of mentalizing in alexithymia. *Neuroimage*, 32(3), 1472-1482.

Mulert, C., Jager, L., Schmitt, R., Bussfeld, P., Pogarell, O., Moller, H. J., et al. (2004). Integration of fMRI and simultaneous EEG: towards a comprehensive understanding of localization and time-course of brain activity in target detection. *Neuroimage*, 22(1), 83-94.

Muller, N. G., & Knight, R. T. (2006). The functional neuroanatomy of working memory: contributions of human brain lesion studies. *Neuroscience*, 139(1), 51-58.

Mummery, C. J., Patterson, K., Price, C. J., Ashburner, J., Frackowiak, R. S., & Hodges, J. R. (2000). A voxel-based morphometry study of semantic dementia: relationship between temporal lobe atrophy and semantic memory. *Ann Neurol*, 47(1), 36-45.

Nadel, L., Campbell, J., & Ryan, L. (2007). Autobiographical Memory Retrieval and Hippocampal Activation as a Function of Repetition and the Passage of Time. *Neural Plast*, 2007, 90472.

Nakamura, K., Honda, M., Okada, T., Hanakawa, T., Toma, K., Fukuyama, H., et al. (2000). Participation of the left posterior inferior temporal cortex in writing and mental recall of kanji orthography: A functional MRI study. *Brain*, 123 (Pt 5), 954-967.

Nakamura, K., Kawashima, R., Sato, N., Nakamura, A., Sugiura, M., Kato, T., et al. (2000). Functional delineation of the human occipito-temporal areas related to face and scene processing. A PET study. *Brain*, 123 (Pt 9), 1903-1912.

Nakamura, W., Anami, K., Mori, T., Saitoh, O., Cichocki, A., & Amari, S. (2006). Removal of ballistocardiogram artifacts from simultaneously recorded EEG and fMRI data using independent component analysis. *IEEE Trans Biomed Eng*, 53(7), 1294-1308.

Navarro, V., Gasto, C., Lomena, F., Mateos, J. J., Marcos, T., & Portella, M. J. (2002). Normalization of frontal cerebral perfusion in remitted elderly major depression: a 12-month follow-up SPECT study. *Neuroimage*, 16(3 Pt 1), 781-787.

Neighbors, B., Kempton, T., & Forehand, R. (1992). Co-occurrence of substance abuse with conduct, anxiety, and depression disorders in juvenile delinquents. *Addict Behav, 17*(4), 379-386.

Nelson, B., Fornito, A., Harrison, B. J., Yucel, M., Sass, L. A., Yung, A. R., et al. (2009). A disturbed sense of self in the psychosis prodrome: linking phenomenology and neurobiology. *Neurosci Biobehav Rev, 33*(6), 807-817.

Nestler, E. J. (2001). Neurobiology. Total recall-the memory of addiction. *Science, 292*(5525), 2266-2267.

Neter, J., Kutner, M., Wasserman, W., & Nachtsheim, C. (2006). *Applied linear statistical models (Fourth ed.).* New York: McGraw Hill/Irwin.

Neumeister, A., Wood, S., Bonne, O., Nugent, A. C., Luckenbaugh, D. A., Young, T., et al. (2005). Reduced hippocampal volume in unmedicated, remitted patients with major depression versus control subjects. *Biol Psychiatry, 57*(8), 935-937.

New, A. S., Hazlett, E. A., Buchsbaum, M. S., Goodman, M., Mitelman, S. A., Newmark, R., et al. (2007). Amygdala-prefrontal disconnection in borderline personality disorder. *Neuropsychopharmacology, 32*(7), 1629-1640.

Nichols, T. E., & Holmes, A. P. (2002). Nonparametric permutation tests for functional neuroimaging: a primer with examples. *Hum Brain Mapp, 15*(1), 1-25.

Nikulina, E. M., Miczek, K. A., & Hammer, R. P., Jr. (2005). Prolonged effects of repeated social defeat stress on mRNA expression and function of mu-opioid receptors in the ventral tegmental area of rats. *Neuropsychopharmacology, 30*(6), 1096-1103.

Nimchinsky, E. A., Vogt, B. A., Morrison, J. H., & Hof, P. R. (1995). Spindle neurons of the human anterior cingulate cortex. *J Comp Neurol, 355*(1), 27-37.

Nitschke, J. B., Sarinopoulos, I., Oathes, D. J., Johnstone, T., Whalen, P. J., Davidson, R. J., et al. (2009). Anticipatory activation in the amygdala and anterior cingulate in generalized anxiety disorder and prediction of treatment response. *Am J Psychiatry, 166*(3), 302-310.

Northoff, G. (2005). Is emotion regulation self-regulation? *Trends Cogn Sci, 9*(9), 408-409; author reply 409-410.

Northoff, G., & Bermpohl, F. (2004). Cortical midline structures and the self. *Trends Cogn Sci, 8*(3), 102-107.

Northoff, G., Heinzel, A., de Greck, M., Bermpohl, F., Dobrowolny, H., & Panksepp, J. (2006). Self-referential processing in our brain--a meta-analysis of imaging studies on the self. *Neuroimage, 31*(1), 440-457.

Northoff, G., Schneider, F., Rotte, M., Matthiae, C., Tempelmann, C., Wiebking, C., et al. (2009). Differential parametric modulation of self-relatedness and emotions in different brain regions. *Hum Brain Mapp, 30*(2), 369-382.

Nowak, S. M., & Marczynski, T. J. (1981). Trait anxiety is reflected in EEG alpha response to stress. *Electroencephalogr Clin Neurophysiol, 52*(2), 175-191.

Nunez, P. L. (1981). A study of origins of the time dependencies of scalp EEG: i--theoretical basis. *IEEE Trans Biomed Eng, 28*(3), 271-280.

Nunez, P. L., Srinivasan, R., Westdorp, A. F., Wijesinghe, R. S., Tucker, D. M., Silberstein, R. B., et al. (1997). EEG coherency. I: Statistics, reference electrode, volume conduction, Laplacians, cortical imaging, and interpretation at multiple scales. *Electroencephalogr Clin Neurophysiol, 103*(5), 499-515.

Nunez, P. L. a. S., R. (2006). *Electric fields of the brain (Second ed.).* New York: Oxford University Press.

Nyberg, L., Marklund, P., Persson, J., Cabeza, R., Forkstam, C., Petersson, K. M., et al. (2003). Common prefrontal activations during working memory, episodic memory, and semantic memory. *Neuropsychologia, 41*(3), 371-377.

Nyberg, L., McIntosh, A. R., Houle, S., Nilsson, L. G., & Tulving, E. (1996). Activation of medial temporal structures during episodic memory retrieval. *Nature, 380*(6576), 715-717.

O'Doherty, J. P., Hampton, A., & Kim, H. (2007). Model-based fMRI and its application to reward learning and decision making. *Ann N Y Acad Sci, 1104*, 35-53.

O'Gorman, R. L., Mehta, M. A., Asherson, P., Zelaya, F. O., Brookes, K. J., Toone, B. K., et al. (2008). Increased cerebral perfusion in adult attention deficit hyperactivity disorder is normalised by stimulant treatment: a non-invasive MRI pilot study. *Neuroimage, 42*(1), 36-41.

Oakes, T. R., Pizzagalli, D. A., Hendrick, A. M., Horras, K. A., Larson, C. L., Abercrombie, H. C., et al. (2004). Functional coupling of simultaneous electrical and metabolic activity in the human brain. *Hum Brain Mapp, 21*(4), 257-270.

Opsomer, R. J., & Guerit, J. M. (1991). [Electric and magnetic brain mapping following stimulation of the dorsal nerve of the penis or clitoris]. *Acta Urol Belg, 59*(1), 63-64.

Osipova, D., Takashima, A., Oostenveld, R., Fernandez, G., Maris, E., & Jensen, O. (2006). Theta and gamma oscillations predict encoding and retrieval of declarative memory. *J Neurosci, 26*(28), 7523-7531.

Overmeyer, S., Bullmore, E. T., Suckling, J., Simmons, A., Williams, S. C., Santosh, P. J., et al. (2001). Distributed grey and white matter deficits in hyperkinetic disorder: MRI evidence for anatomical abnormality in an attentional network. *Psychol Med, 31*(8), 1425-1435.

Ovtscharoff, W., Jr., Helmeke, C., & Braun, K. (2006). Lack of paternal care affects synaptic development in the anterior cingulate cortex. *Brain Res, 1116*(1), 58-63.

Oya, H., Adolphs, R., Kawasaki, H., Bechara, A., Damasio, A., & Howard, M. A., 3rd (2005). Electrophysiological correlates of reward prediction error recorded in the human prefrontal cortex. *Proc Natl Acad Sci U S A, 102*(23), 8351-8356.

Ozcan, M., Baumgartner, U., Vucurevic, G., Stoeter, P., & Treede, R. D. (2005). Spatial resolution of fMRI in the human parasylvian cortex: comparison of somatosensory and auditory activation. *Neuroimage*, 25(3), 877-887.

Pagnoni, G., Zink, C. F., Montague, P. R., & Berns, G. S. (2002). Activity in human ventral striatum locked to errors of reward prediction. *Nat Neurosci*, 5(2), 97-98.

Pang, E. W., Wang, F., Malone, M., Kadis, D. S., & Donner, E. J. (2011). Localization of Broca's area using verb generation tasks in the MEG: Validation against fMRI. *Neurosci Lett,* 490(3), 215-219.

Panksepp, J. (2003). At the interface of the affective, behavioral, and cognitive neurosciences: decoding the emotional feelings of the brain. *Brain Cogn*, 52(1), 4-14.

Panksepp, J. (2005). Affective consciousness: Core emotional feelings in animals and humans. *Conscious Cogn*, 14(1), 30-80.

Panksepp, J., & Northoff, G. (2009). The trans-species core SELF: the emergence of active cultural and neuro-ecological agents through self-related processing within subcortical-cortical midline networks. *Conscious Cogn*, 18(1), 193-215.

Paquette, V., Beauregard, M., Beaulieu-Prevost, D. (2009). Effect of a psychoneurotherapy on brain electromagnetic tomography in individuals with major depressive disorder. Psychiatry Research: *Neuroimaging*.174:231-239

Paquette, V., Levesque, J., Mensour, B., Leroux, J. M., Beaudoin, G., Bourgouin, P., et al. (2003). "Change the mind and you change the brain": effects of cognitive-behavioral therapy on the neural correlates of spider phobia. *Neuroimage*, 18(2), 401-409.

Pardo, J. V., Fox, P. T., & Raichle, M. E. (1991). Localization of a human system for sustained attention by positron emission tomography. *Nature*, 349(6304), 61-64.

Parker, S. T., Mitchell, R.W., Boccia, M.L. (1994). *Self-awareness in Animals and Humans*. New York: Cambridge University Press.

Pascual-Marqui, R. D. (2002). Standardized low-resolution brain electromagnetic tomography (sLORETA): technical details. *Methods Find Exp Clin Pharmacol*, 24 Suppl D, 5-12.

Pascual-Marqui, R. D., & Biscay-Lirio, R. (1993). Spatial resolution of neuronal generators based on EEG and MEG measurements. Int J Neurosci, 68(1-2), 93-105.

Pascual-Marqui, R. D., Esslen, M., Kochi, K., & Lehmann, D. (2002). Functional imaging with low-resolution brain electromagnetic tomography (LORETA): a review. Methods *Find Exp Clin Pharmacol,* 24 Suppl C, 91-95.

Pascual-Marqui, R. D., Gonzalez-Andino, S. L., Valdes-Sosa, P. A., & Biscay-Lirio, R. (1988). Current source density estimation and interpolation based on the spherical harmonic Fourier expansion. *Int J Neurosci*, 43(3-4), 237-249.

Pascual-Marqui, R. D., & Lehmann, D. (1993a). Comparison of topographic maps and the reference electrode: comments on two papers by Desmedt and collaborators. *Electroencephalogr Clin Neurophysiol*, 88(6), 530-531, 534-536.

Pascual-Marqui, R. D., & Lehmann, D. (1993b). Topographic maps, source localization inference, and the reference electrode: comments on a paper by Desmedt et al. *Electroencephalogr Clin Neurophysiol*, 88(6), 532-536.

Pascual-Marqui, R. D., Lehmann, D., Koenig, T., Kochi, K., Merlo, M. C., Hell, D., et al. (1999). Low resolution brain electromagnetic tomography (LORETA) functional imaging in acute, neuroleptic-naive, first-episode, productive schizophrenia. *Psychiatry Res*, 90(3), 169-179.

Pascual-Marqui, R. D., Michel, C. M., & Lehmann, D. (1994). Low resolution electromagnetic tomography: a new method for localizing electrical activity in the brain. *Int J Psychophysiol*, 18(1), 49-65.

Pascual-Marqui, R. D., Michel, C. M., & Lehmann, D. (1995). Segmentation of brain electrical activity into microstates: model estimation and validation. *IEEE Trans Biomed Eng*, 42(7), 658-665.

Pascual-Marqui, R. D., Valdes-Sosa, P. A., & Alvarez-Amador, A. (1988). A parametric model for multichannel EEG spectra. *Int J Neurosci*, 40(1-2), 89-99.

Pascual-Montano, A., Taylor, K. A., Winkler, H., Pascual-Marqui, R. D., & Carazo, J. M. (2002). Quantitative self-organizing maps for clustering electron tomograms. *J Struct Biol*, 138(1-2), 114-122.

Pascual Marqui, R. D. (1999). Review of methods for solving the EEG inverse problem. *International Journal of Bioelectromagnetism*, 1, 75 - 86.

Paulesu, E., Frith, C. D., & Frackowiak, R. S. (1993). The neural correlates of the verbal component of working memory. *Nature*, 362(6418), 342-345.

Paulus, M. P., Feinstein, J. S., Leland, D., & Simmons, A. N. (2005). Superior temporal gyrus and insula provide response and outcome-dependent information during assessment and action selection in a decision-making situation. *Neuroimage*, 25(2), 607-615.

Peniston, E. G., & Kulkosky, P. J. (1989). Alpha-theta brainwave training and beta-endorphin levels in alcoholics. *Alcohol Clin Exp Res*, 13(2), 271-279.

Pennington, K., Dicker, P., Dunn, M. J., & Cotter, D. R. (2008). Proteomic analysis reveals protein changes within layer 2 of the insular cortex in schizophrenia. *Proteomics*, 8(23-24), 5097-5107.

Pennington, K., Dicker, P., Hudson, L., & Cotter, D. R. (2008). Evidence for reduced neuronal somal size within the insular cortex in schizophrenia, but not in affective disorders. *Schizophr Res*, 106(2-3), 164-171.

Peterson, B. S., Potenza, M. N., Wang, Z., Zhu, H., Martin, A., Marsh, R., et al. (2009). An FMRI study of the effects of psychostimulants on default-mode processing during Stroop task performance in youths with ADHD. *Am J Psychiatry*, 166(11), 1286-1294.

Petersson, K. M., Nichols, T. E., Poline, J. B., & Holmes, A. P. (1999). Statistical limitations in functional neuroimaging. II. Signal detection and statistical inference. *Philos Trans R Soc Lond B Biol Sci*, 354(1387), 1261-1281.

Petsche, H., Lacroix, D., Lindner, K., Rappelsberger, P., & Schmidt-Henrich, E. (1992). Thinking with images or thinking with language: a pilot EEG probability mapping study. *Int J Psychophysiol*, 12(1), 31-39.

Phan, K. L., Fitzgerald, D. A., Nathan, P. J., Moore, G. J., Uhde, T. W., & Tancer, M. E. (2005). Neural substrates for voluntary suppression of negative affect: a functional magnetic resonance imaging study. *Biol Psychiatry*, 57(3), 210-219.

Phan, K. L., Liberzon, I., Welsh, R. C., Britton, J. C., & Taylor, S. F. (2003). Habituation of rostral anterior cingulate cortex to repeated emotionally salient pictures. *Neuropsychopharmacology*, 28(7), 1344-1350.

Phan, K. L., Wager, T., Taylor, S. F., & Liberzon, I. (2002). Functional neuroanatomy of emotion: a meta-analysis of emotion activation studies in PET and fMRI. *Neuroimage*, 16(2), 331-348.

Phillips, C., Rugg, M. D., & Fristont, K. J. (2002). Systematic regularization of linear inverse solutions of the EEG source localization problem. *Neuroimage*, 17(1), 287-301.

Pienkowski, M., Munguia, R., & Eggermont, J. J. (2011). Passive exposure of adult cats to bandlimited tone pip ensembles or noise leads to long-term response suppression in auditory cortex. *Hear Res.* 277:117-126

Pizzagalli, D., Pascual-Marqui, R. D., Nitschke, J. B., Oakes, T. R., Larson, C. L., Abercrombie, H. C., et al. (2001). Anterior cingulate activity as a predictor of degree of treatment response in major depression: evidence from brain electrical tomography analysis. *Am J Psychiatry*, 158(3), 405-415.

Pizzagalli, D. A., Bogdan, R., Ratner, K. G., & Jahn, A. L. (2007). Increased perceived stress is associated with blunted hedonic capacity: potential implications for depression research. *Behav Res Ther*, 45(11), 2742-2753.

Pizzagalli, D. A., Goetz, E., Ostacher, M., Iosifescu, D. V., & Perlis, R. H. (2008). Euthymic patients with bipolar disorder show decreased reward learning in a probabilistic reward task. *Biol Psychiatry*, 64(2), 162-168.

Pizzagalli, D. A., Lehmann, D., Hendrick, A. M., Regard, M., Pascual-Marqui, R. D., & Davidson, R. J. (2002). Affective judgments of faces modulate early activity (approximately 160 ms) within the fusiform gyri. *Neuroimage*, 16(3 Pt 1), 663-677.

Pizzagalli, D. A., Nitschke, J. B., Oakes, T. R., Hendrick, A. M., Horras, K. A., Larson, C. L., et al. (2002). Brain electrical tomography in depression: the importance of symptom severity, anxiety, and melancholic features. *Biol Psychiatry*, 52(2), 73-85.

Pizzagalli, D. A., Oakes, T. R., & Davidson, R. J. (2003). Coupling of theta activity and glucose metabolism in the human rostral anterior cingulate cortex: an EEG/PET study of normal and depressed subjects. *Psychophysiology*, 40(6), 939-949.

Pizzagalli, D. A., Sherwood, R. J., Henriques, J. B., & Davidson, R. J. (2005). Frontal brain asymmetry and reward responsiveness: a source-localization study. *Psychol Sci,* 16(10), 805-813.

Poldrack, R. A. (2002). Neural systems for perceptual skill learning. *Behav Cogn Neurosci Rev*, 1(1), 76-83.

Poldrack, R. A., Desmond, J. E., Glover, G. H., & Gabrieli, J. D. (1998). The neural basis of visual skill learning: an fMRI study of mirror reading. *Cereb Cortex*, 8(1), 1-10.

Poldrack, R. A., & Gabrieli, J. D. (2001). Characterizing the neural mechanisms of skill learning and repetition priming: evidence from mirror reading. *Brain*, 124(Pt 1), 67-82.

Poldrack, R. A., Selco, S. L., Field, J. E., & Cohen, N. J. (1999). The relationship between skill learning and repetition priming: experimental and computational analyses. *J Exp Psychol Learn Mem Cogn*, 25(1), 208-235.

Pollock, V. E. (1992). Meta-analysis of subjective sensitivity to alcohol in sons of alcoholics. A*m J Psychiatry,* 149(11), 1534-1538.

Pollock, V. E., & Schneider, L. S. (1990). Quantitative, waking EEG research on depression. *Biol Psychiatry,* 27(7), 757-780.

Polunina, A. G., & Davydov, D. M. (2006). EEG correlates of Wechsler Adult Intelligence Scale. *Int J Neurosci*, 116(10), 1231-1248.

Posner, M. I. (1994). Attention: the mechanisms of consciousness. *Proc Natl Acad Sci U S A*, 91(16), 7398-7403.

Posner, M. I., & Dehaene, S. (1994). Attentional networks. *Trends Neurosci*, 17(2), 75-79.

Posner, M. I., & Rothbart, M. K. (1998). Attention, self-regulation and consciousness. *Philos Trans R Soc Lond B Biol Sci*, 353(1377), 1915-1927.

Potenza, M. N. (2007). To do or not to do? The complexities of addiction, motivation, self-control, and impulsivity. *Am J Psychiatry*, 164(1), 4-6.

Potvin, S., Stip, E., Lipp, O., Roy, M. A., Demers, M. F., Bouchard, R. H., et al. (2008). Anhedonia and social adaptation predict substance abuse evolution in dual diagnosis schizophrenia. *Am J Drug Alcohol Abuse*, 34(1), 75-82.

Prasad, N. G. N., Rao, J.N.K. (1990). The Estimation of the Mean Squared Error of Small-Area Estimators. *Journal of the American Statistical Association*, 85(409), 163-171.

Prichep, L. S., Alper, K. R., Kowalik, S. C., Vaysblat, L. S., Merkin, H. A., Tom, M., et al. (1999). Prediction of treatment outcome in cocaine dependent males using quantitative EEG. *Drug Alcohol Depend*, 54(1), 35-43.

Prichep, L. S., Alper, K. R., Sverdlov, L., Kowalik, S. C., John, E. R., Merkin, H., et al. (2002). Outcome related electrophysiological subtypes of cocaine dependence. *Clin Electroencephalogr,* 33(1), 8-20.

Prichep, L. S., Kowalik, S. C., Alper, K., & de Jesus, C. (1995). Quantitative EEG characteristics of children exposed in utero to cocaine. *Clin Electroencephalogr,* 26(3), 166-172.

Pruessner, J. C., Dedovic, K., Khalili-Mahani, N., Engert, V., Pruessner, M., Buss, C., et al. (2008). Deactivation of the limbic system during acute psychosocial stress: evidence from positron emission tomography and functional magnetic resonance imaging studies. *Biol Psychiatry*, 63(2), 234-240.

Pruessner, J. C., Dedovic, K., Pruessner, M., Lord, C., Buss, C., Collins, L., et al. Stress regulation in the central nervous system: evidence from structural and functional neuroimaging studies in human populations - 2008 Curt Richter Award Winner. *Psychoneuroendocrinology,* 35(1), 179-191.

Pruessner, J. C., Gaab, J., Hellhammer, D. H., Lintz, D., Schommer, N., & Kirschbaum, C. (1997). Increasing correlations between personality traits and cortisol stress responses obtained by data aggregation. *Psychoneuroendocrinology*, 22(8), 615-625.

Pruessner, J. C., Hellhammer, D. H., & Kirschbaum, C. (1999). Burnout, perceived stress, and cortisol responses to awakening. *Psychosom Med*, 61(2), 197-204.

Pruessner, M., Hellhammer, D. H., Pruessner, J. C., & Lupien, S. J. (2003). Self-reported depressive symptoms and stress levels in healthy young men: associations with the cortisol response to awakening. *Psychosom Med*, 65(1), 92-99.

Quintana, H., Snyder, S. M., Purnell, W., Aponte, C., & Sita, J. (2007). Comparison of a standard psychiatric evaluation to rating scales and EEG in the differential diagnosis of attention-deficit/hyperactivity disorder. *Psychiatry Res*, 152(2-3), 211-222.

Raichle, M. E. (1998). Behind the scenes of functional brain imaging: a historical and physiological perspective. Proc Natl Acad Sci U S A, 95(3), 765-772.

Raichle, M. E., MacLeod, A. M., Snyder, A. Z., Powers, W. J., Gusnard, D. A., & Shulman, G. L. (2001). A default mode of brain function. Proc Natl Acad Sci U S A, 98(2), 676-682.

Raichle, M. E., & Snyder, A. Z. (2007). A default mode of brain function: a brief history of an evolving idea. Neuroimage, 37(4), 1083-1090; discussion 1097-1089.

Ramachandran, V. S. (1995). Anosognosia in parietal lobe syndrome. Conscious Cogn, 4(1), 22-51.

Ramnani, N., & Miall, R. C. (2004). A system in the human brain for predicting the actions of others. Nat Neurosci, 7(1), 85-90.

Ramnani, N., & Owen, A. M. (2004). Anterior prefrontal cortex: insights into function from anatomy and neuroimaging. Nat Rev Neurosci, 5(3), 184-194.

Rappelsberger, P. (1989). The reference problem and mapping of coherence: a simulation study. Brain Topogr, 2(1-2), 63-72.

Rauch, S. L., Jenike, M. A., Alpert, N. M., Baer, L., Breiter, H. C., Savage, C. R., et al. (1994). Regional cerebral blood flow measured during symptom provocation in obsessive-compulsive disorder using oxygen 15-labeled carbon dioxide and positron emission tomography. Arch Gen Psychiatry, 51(1), 62-70.

Ravindran, A. V., Smith, A., Cameron, C., Bhatla, R., Cameron, I., Georgescu, T. M., et al. (2009). Toward a functional neuroanatomy of dysthymia: A functional magnetic resonance imaging study. Journal of Affective Disorders, 119(1-3), 9-15.

Ray, W. J., & Cole, H. W. (1985). EEG alpha activity reflects attentional demands, and beta activity reflects emotional and cognitive processes. Science, 228(4700), 750-752.

Regier, D. A., Farmer, M. E., Rae, D. S., Locke, B. Z., Keith, S. J., Judd, L. L., et al. (1990). Comorbidity of mental disorders with alcohol and other drug abuse. Results from the Epidemiologic Catchment Area (ECA) Study. JAMA, 264(19), 2511-2518.

Resnick, S. M., Driscoll, I., & Lamar, M. (2007). Vulnerability of the Orbitofrontal Cortex to Age-Associated Structural and Functional Brain Changes. Ann N Y Acad Sci.1121:562-575

Ricardo-Garcell, J., Gonzalez-Olvera, J. J., Miranda, E., Harmony, T., Reyes, E., Almeida, L., et al. (2009). EEG sources in a group of patients with major depressive disorders. Int J Psychophysiol, 71(1), 70-74.

Rilling, J. K., Barks, S. K., Parr, L. A., Preuss, T. M., Faber, T. L., Pagnoni, G., et al. (2007). A comparison of resting-state brain activity in humans and chimpanzees. Proc Natl Acad Sci U S A, 104(43), 17146-17151.

Robbins, T. W., & Everitt, B. J. (2002). Limbic-striatal memory systems and drug addiction. Neurobiol Learn Mem, 78(3), 625-636.

Roemer, R. A., Cornwell, A., Dewart, D., Jackson, P., & Ercegovac, D. V. (1995). Quantitative electroencephalographic analyses in cocaine-preferring polysubstance abusers during abstinence. Psychiatry Res, 58(3), 247-257.

Rolls, E. T., Critchley, H. D., Browning, A. S., Hernadi, I., & Lenard, L. (1999). Responses to the sensory properties of fat of neurons in the primate orbitofrontal cortex. J Neurosci, 19(4), 1532-1540.

Rosen, M. R., & Robinson, R. B. (1990). Developmental changes in alpha adrenergic modulation of ventricular pacemaker function. Ann N Y Acad Sci, 588, 137-144.

Rosenberg, R. N., Pleasure, D.E. (1998). *Comprehensive Neurology (Second ed.).* New York: Wiley-Liss.

Rosenblatt, A. D., & Thickstun, J. T. (1977). Affect, emotion, and activation theories. *Psychol Issues,* 11(2-3), 194-217.

Rosso, I. M. (2005). Review: hippocampal volume is reduced in people with unipolar depression. *Evid Based Ment Health,* 8(2), 45.

Rozin, P., & Fallon, A. E. (1987). A perspective on disgust. *Psychol Rev,* 94(1), 23-41.

Rubia, K. (2002). The dynamic approach to neurodevelopmental psychiatric disorders: use of fMRI combined with neuropsychology to elucidate the dynamics of psychiatric disorders, exemplified in ADHD and schizophrenia. *Behav Brain Res,* 130(1-2), 47-56.

Rubia, K., Russell, T., Overmeyer, S., Brammer, M. J., Bullmore, E. T., Sharma, T., et al. (2001). Mapping motor inhibition: conjunctive brain activations across different versions of go/no-go and stop tasks. *Neuroimage,* 13(2), 250-261.

Rubia, K., Smith, A. B., Taylor, E., & Brammer, M. (2007). Linear age-correlated functional development of right inferior fronto-striato-cerebellar networks during response inhibition and anterior cingulate during error-related processes. *Hum Brain Mapp.* 28:1163-1177

Sabbagh, M. A., & Flynn, J. (2006). Mid-frontal EEG alpha asymmetries predict individual differences in one aspect of theory of mind: mental state decoding. *Soc Neurosci,* 1(3-4), 299-308.

Sahay, A., & Hen, R. (2007). Adult hippocampal neurogenesis in depression. *Nat Neurosci,* 10(9), 1110-1115.

Sala, M., Perez, J., Soloff, P., Ucelli di Nemi, S., Caverzasi, E., Soares, J. C., et al. (2004). Stress and hippocampal abnormalities in psychiatric disorders. *Eur Neuropsychopharmacol,* 14(5), 393-405.

Salamone, J. D. (1994). The involvement of nucleus accumbens dopamine in appetitive and aversive motivation. *Behav Brain Res,* 61(2), 117-133.

Saletu-Zyhlarz, G. M., Arnold, O., Anderer, P., Oberndorfer, S., Walter, H., Lesch, O. M., et al. (2004). Differences in brain function between relapsing and abstaining alcohol-dependent patients, evaluated by EEG mapping. *Alcohol Alcohol,* 39(3), 233-240.

Saletu, B., Anderer, P., Di Padova, C., Assandri, A., & Saletu-Zyhlarz, G. M. (2002). Electrophysiological neuroimaging of the central effects of S-adenosyl-L-methionine by mapping of electroencephalograms and event-related potentials and low-resolution brain electromagnetic tomography. *Am J Clin Nutr,* 76(5), 1162S-1171S.

Saletu, B., Anderer, P., Saletu-Zyhlarz, G. M., & Pascual-Marqui, R. D. (2002). EEG topography and tomography in diagnosis and treatment of mental disorders: evidence for a key-lock principle. *Methods Find Exp Clin Pharmacol,* 24 Suppl D, 97-106.

Saletu, B., Saletu-Zyhlarz, G., Anderer, P., Brandstatter, N., Frey, R., Gruber, G., et al. (1997). Nonorganic insomnia in generalized anxiety disorder. 2. Comparative studies on sleep, awakening, daytime vigilance and anxiety under lorazepam plus diphenhydramine (Somnium) versus lorazepam alone, utilizing clinical, polysomnographic and EEG mapping methods. *Neuropsychobiology,* 36(3), 130-152.

Salomons, T. V., Johnstone, T., Backonja, M. M., & Davidson, R. J. (2004). Perceived controllability modulates the neural response to pain. *J Neurosci,* 24(32), 7199-7203.

Sambataro, F., Murty, V. P., Callicott, J. H., Tan, H. Y., Das, S., Weinberger, D. R., et al. (2008). Age-related alterations in default mode network: Impact on working memory performance. *Neurobiol Aging.* 31:839-852

Sanei, S. C., J.A. (2007). *EEG Signal Processing.* West Sussex: John Wiley & Sons, Ltd.

Santesso, D. L., Steele, K. T., Bogdan, R., Holmes, A. J., Deveney, C. M., Meites, T. M., et al. (2008). Enhanced negative feedback responses in remitted depression. *Neuroreport,* 19(10), 1045-1048.

Sapolsky, R. M. (2004). Organismal stress and telomeric aging: an unexpected connection. *Proc Natl Acad Sci U S A,* 101(50), 17323-17324.

Sartori, G., Snitz, B. E., Sorcinelli, L., & Daum, I. (2004). Remote memory in advanced Alzheimer's disease. *Arch Clin Neuropsychol,* 19(6), 779-789.

Sarvas, J. (1987). Basic mathematical and electromagnetic concepts of the biomagnetic inverse problem. *Phys Med Biol,* 32(1), 11-22.

Satoh, T., Nakai, S., Sato, T., & Kimura, M. (2003). Correlated coding of motivation and outcome of decision by dopamine neurons. *J Neurosci,* 23(30), 9913-9923.

Sauseng, P., Klimesch, W., Doppelmayr, M., Pecherstorfer, T., Freunberger, R., & Hanslmayr, S. (2005). EEG alpha synchronization and functional coupling during top-down processing in a working memory task. *Hum Brain Mapp,* 26(2), 148-155.

Sauseng, P., Klimesch, W., Freunberger, R., Pecherstorfer, T., Hanslmayr, S., & Doppelmayr, M. (2006). Relevance of EEG alpha and theta oscillations during task switching. *Exp Brain Res,* 170(3), 295-301.

Sauseng, P., Klimesch, W., Schabus, M., & Doppelmayr, M. (2005). Fronto-parietal EEG coherence in theta and upper alpha reflect central executive functions of working memory. *Int J Psychophysiol,* 57(2), 97-103.

Sauseng, P., Klimesch, W., Stadler, W., Schabus, M., Doppelmayr, M., Hanslmayr, S., et al. (2005). A shift of visual spatial attention is selectively associated with human EEG alpha activity. *Eur J Neurosci,* 22(11), 2917-2926.

Sawamoto, N., Honda, M., Okada, T., Hanakawa, T., Kanda, M., Fukuyama, H., et al. (2000). Expectation of pain enhances responses to nonpainful somatosensory stimulation in the anterior cingulate cortex and parietal operculum/posterior insula: an event-related functional magnetic resonance imaging study. *J Neurosci,* 20(19), 7438-7445.

Saxena, S., Brody, A. L., Schwartz, J. M., & Baxter, L. R. (1998). Neuroimaging and frontal-subcortical circuitry in obsessive-compulsive disorder. *Br J Psychiatry Suppl*(35), 26-37.

Schadwinkel, S., & Gutschalk, A. (2011). Transient BOLD activity locked to perceptual reversals of auditory streaming in human auditory cortex and inferior colliculus. *J Neurophysiol.* 105:1197-1983

Schafer, R. (1973). Concepts of self and identity and the experience of separation-individuation in adolescence. *Psychoanal Q,* 42(1), 42-59.

Scheres, A., Lee, A., & Sumiya, M. (2008). Temporal reward discounting and ADHD: task and symptom specific effects. *J Neural Transm,* 115(2), 221-226.

Scheres, A., Milham, M. P., Knutson, B., & Castellanos, F. X. (2007). Ventral striatal hyporesponsiveness during reward anticipation in attention-deficit/hyperactivity disorder. *Biol Psychiatry,* 61(5), 720-724.

Scherg, M. (1994). From EEG source localization to source imaging. *Acta Neurol Scand Suppl,* 152, 29-30.

Scherg, M., & Ebersole, J. S. (1994). Brain source imaging of focal and multifocal epileptiform EEG activity. *Neurophysiol Clin,* 24(1), 51-60.

Scherg, M., Ille, N., Bornfleth, H., & Berg, P. (2002). Advanced tools for digital EEG review: virtual source montages, whole-head mapping, correlation, and phase analysis. *J Clin Neurophysiol,* 19(2), 91-112.

Schienle, A., Schafer, A., Stark, R., Walter, B., & Vaitl, D. (2005a). Gender differences in the processing of disgust- and fear-inducing pictures: an fMRI study. *Neuroreport,* 16(3), 277-280.

Schienle, A., Schafer, A., Stark, R., Walter, B., & Vaitl, D. (2005b). Neural responses of OCD patients towards disorder-relevant, generally disgust-inducing and fear-inducing pictures. *Int J Psychophysiol,* 57(1), 69-77.

Schienle, A., Schafer, A., Stark, R., Walter, B., & Vaitl, D. (2005c). Relationship between disgust sensitivity, trait anxiety and brain activity during disgust induction. *Neuropsychobiology,* 51(2), 86-92.

Schmid, R. G., Tirsch, W. S., & Scherb, H. (2002). Correlation between spectral EEG parameters and intelligence test variables in school-age children. *Clin Neurophysiol,* 113(10), 1647-1656.

Schonberg, T., Daw, N. D., Joel, D., & O'Doherty, J. P. (2007). Reinforcement learning signals in the human striatum distinguish learners from nonlearners during reward-based decision making. *J Neurosci, 27*(47), 12860-12867.

Schumann, J., Michaeli, A., & Yaka, R. (2009). Src-protein tyrosine kinases are required for cocaine-induced increase in the expression and function of the NMDA receptor in the ventral tegmental area. *J Neurochem, 108*(3), 697-706.

Schwartz, J. M. (1998). Neuroanatomical aspects of cognitive-behavioural therapy response in obsessive-compulsive disorder. An evolving perspective on brain and behaviour. *Br J Psychiatry Suppl*(35), 38-44.

Schwartz, J. M., Stoessel, P. W., Baxter, L. R., Jr., Martin, K. M., & Phelps, M. E. (1996). Systematic changes in cerebral glucose metabolic rate after successful behavior modification treatment of obsessive-compulsive disorder. *Arch Gen Psychiatry, 53*(2), 109-113.

Schwarz, E. D., & Perry, B. D. (1994). The post-traumatic response in children and adolescents. *Psychiatr Clin North Am, 17*(2), 311-326.

Schweitzer, J. B., Faber, T. L., Grafton, S. T., Tune, L. E., Hoffman, J. M., & Kilts, C. D. (2000). Alterations in the functional anatomy of working memory in adult attention deficit hyperactivity disorder. *Am J Psychiatry, 157*(2), 278-280.

Seidman, L. J., Valera, E. M., & Bush, G. (2004). Brain function and structure in adults with attention-deficit/hyperactivity disorder. *Psychiatr Clin North Am, 27*(2), 323-347.

Seidman, L. J., Valera, E. M., & Makris, N. (2005). Structural brain imaging of attention-deficit/hyperactivity disorder. *Biol Psychiatry, 57*(11), 1263-1272.

Seidman, L. J., Valera, E. M., Makris, N., Monuteaux, M. C., Boriel, D. L., Kelkar, K., et al. (2006). Dorsolateral prefrontal and anterior cingulate cortex volumetric abnormalities in adults with attention-deficit/hyperactivity disorder identified by magnetic resonance imaging. *Biol Psychiatry, 60*(10), 1071-1080.

Sekihara, K., Sahani, M., & Nagarajan, S. S. (2005). Localization bias and spatial resolution of adaptive and non-adaptive spatial filters for MEG source reconstruction. *Neuroimage, 25*(4), 1056-1067.

Sekihara, K., Sahani, M., & Nagarajan, S. S. (2005). Localization bias and spatial resolution of adaptive and non-adaptive spatial filters for MEG source reconstruction. *Neuroimage, 25*(4), 1056-1067.

Seminowicz, D. A., Mayberg, H. S., McIntosh, A. R., Goldapple, K., Kennedy, S., Segal, Z., et al. (2004). Limbic-frontal circuitry in major depression: a path modeling metanalysis. *Neuroimage, 22*(1), 409-418.

Shah, S. G., Klumpp, H., Angstadt, M., Nathan, P. J., & Phan, K. L. (2009). Amygdala and insula response to emotional images in patients with generalized social anxiety disorder. *J Psychiatry Neurosci, 34*(4), 296-302.

Shankaranarayana Rao, B. S., Raju, T. R., & Meti, B. L. (1998). Self-stimulation of lateral hypothalamus and ventral tegmentum increases the levels of noradrenaline, dopamine, glutamate, and AChE activity, but not 5-hydroxytryptamine and GABA levels in hippocampus and motor cortex. *Neurochem Res*, 23(8), 1053-1059.

Sheehan, M. F. (1993). Dual diagnosis. *Psychiatr Q,* 64(2), 107-134.

Sheline, Y. I., Barch, D. M., Price, J. L., Rundle, M. M., Vaishnavi, S. N., Snyder, A. Z., et al. (2009). The default mode network and self-referential processes in depression. *Proc Natl Acad Sci U S A*, 106(6), 1942-1947.

Sherlin, L., Budzynski, T., Kogan Budzynski, H., Congedo, M., Fischer, M. E., & Buchwald, D. (2007). Low-resolution electromagnetic brain tomography (LORETA) of monozygotic twins discordant for chronic fatigue syndrome. *Neuroimage*, 34(4), 1438-1442.

Shigemura, S., Nishimura, T., Tsubai, M., & Yokoi, H. (2004). An investigation of EEG artifacts elimination using a neural network with non-recursive 2nd order volterra filters. Conf Proc *IEEE Eng Med Biol Soc*, 1, 612-615.

Shulman, G. L., Corbetta, M., Buckner, R. L., Raichle, M. E., Fiez, J. A., Miezin, F. M., et al. (1997). Top-down modulation of early sensory cortex. *Cereb Cortex*, 7(3), 193-206.

Shulman, G. L., Ollinger, J. M., Akbudak, E., Conturo, T. E., Snyder, A. Z., Petersen, S. E., et al. (1999). Areas involved in encoding and applying directional expectations to moving objects. *J Neurosci*, 19(21), 9480-9496.

Shulman, G. L., Ollinger, J. M., Linenweber, M., Petersen, S. E., & Corbetta, M. (2001). Multiple neural correlates of detection in the human brain. *Proc Natl Acad Sci U S A,* 98(1), 313-318.

Shulman, G. L., Schwarz, J., Miezin, F. M., & Petersen, S. E. (1998). Effect of motion contrast on human cortical responses to moving stimuli. J *Neurophysiol*, 79(5), 2794-2803.

Silk, T., Vance, A., Rinehart, N., Egan, G., O'Boyle, M., Bradshaw, J. L., et al. (2005). Fronto-parietal activation in attention-deficit hyperactivity disorder, combined type: functional magnetic resonance imaging study. *Br J Psychiatry*, 187, 282-283.

Silk, T. J., Vance, A., Rinehart, N., Bradshaw, J. L., & Cunnington, R. (2009). White-matter abnormalities in attention deficit hyperactivity disorder: a diffusion tensor imaging study. *Hum Brain Mapp*, 30(9), 2757-2765.

Singer, L. T., Eisengart, L. J., Minnes, S., Noland, J., Jey, A., Lane, C., et al. (2005). Prenatal cocaine exposure and infant cognition. *Infant Behav Dev*, 28(4), 431-444.

Sinha, R., Catapano, D., & O'Malley, S. (1999). Stress-induced craving and stress response in cocaine dependent individuals. *Psychopharmacology (Berl)*, 142(4), 343-351.

Smit, D. J., Posthuma, D., Boomsma, D. I., & De Geus, E. J. (2007). The relation between frontal EEG asymmetry and the risk for anxiety and depression. *Biol Psychol*, 74(1), 26-33.

Smith, L. C. (2001). Dual diagnosis. Effective recognition and management of severe mental illness and substance abuse. *JAAPA*, 14(2), 22-24, 27-30, 35-26 passim.

Smythies, J. R. (1966). *The Neurological Foundations of Psychiatry*. New York: Academic Press.

Smythies, J. R., & Sykes, E. A. (1966). Structure-activity relationship studies on mescaline: the effect of dimethoxyphenylethylamine and N:N-dimethyl mescaline on the conditioned avoidance response in the rat. *Psychopharmacologia*, 8(5), 324-330.

Sokhadze, T. M., Cannon, R. L., & Trudeau, D. L. (2008). EEG Biofeedback as a treatment for substance use disorders: Review, rating of efficacy and recommendations for further research. *Journal of Neurotherapy: Investigations in Neuromodulation, Neurofeedback and Applied Neuroscience,* 12(1), 5 - 43.

Soliman, A., O'Driscoll, G. A., Pruessner, J., Holahan, A. L., Boileau, I., Gagnon, D., et al. (2008). Stress-induced dopamine release in humans at risk of psychosis: a [11C]raclopride PET study. *Neuropsychopharmacology,* 33(8), 2033-2041.

Sonuga-Barke, E. J., Taylor, E., & Heptinstall, E. (1992). Hyperactivity and delay aversion--II. The effect of self versus externally imposed stimulus presentation periods on memory. *J Child Psychol Psychiatry,* 33(2), 399-409.

Sonuga-Barke, E. J., Taylor, E., Sembi, S., & Smith, J. (1992). Hyperactivity and delay aversion--I. The effect of delay on choice. *J Child Psychol Psychiatry,* 33(2), 387-398.

Sparks, D. L. (2002). The brainstem control of saccadic eye movements. *Nat Rev Neurosci*, 3(12), 952-964.

Spencer, T. J., Biederman, J., & Mick, E. (2007). Attention-deficit/hyperactivity disorder: diagnosis, lifespan, comorbidities, and neurobiology. *J Pediatr Psychol,* 32(6), 631-642.

Sperling, R. A., Laviolette, P. S., O'Keefe, K., O'Brien, J., Rentz, D. M., Pihlajamaki, M., et al. (2009). Amyloid deposition is associated with impaired default network function in older persons without dementia. *Neuron,* 63(2), 178-188.

Spironelli, C., Penolazzi, B., & Angrilli, A. (2008). Dysfunctional hemispheric asymmetry of theta and beta EEG activity during linguistic tasks in developmental dyslexia. *Biol Psychol,* 77(2), 123-131.

Sridharan, D., Levitin, D. J., & Menon, V. (2008). A critical role for the right fronto-insular cortex in switching between central-executive and default-mode networks. *Proc Natl Acad Sci U S A*, 105(34), 12569-12574.

Staiman, K. E. (1998). Insights into temporal lobe function and its relationship to the visual system. *Clinical Eye and Vision Care*, 10, 119 - 124.

Stanwood, G. D., & Levitt, P. (2001). Prenatal cocaine exposure as a risk factor for later developmental outcomes. *JAMA*, 286(1), 45; author reply 46-47.

Stanwood, G. D., Washington, R. A., & Levitt, P. (2001). Identification of a sensitive period of prenatal cocaine exposure that alters the development of the anterior cingulate cortex. *Cereb Cortex*, 11(5), 430-440.

Steriade, M. (2004). Slow-wave sleep: serotonin, neuronal plasticity, and seizures. *Arch Ital Biol*, 142(4), 359-367.

Steriade, M., Gloor, P., Llinas, R. R., Lopes de Silva, F. H., & Mesulam, M. M. (1990). Basic mechanisms of cerebral rhythmic activities. *Electroencephalography and Clinical Neurophysiology*, 76, 481-508.

Stevens, M. C., Pearlson, G. D., & Kiehl, K. A. (2007). An FMRI auditory oddball study of combined-subtype attention deficit hyperactivity disorder. *Am J Psychiatry*, 164(11), 1737-1749.

Steyn-Ross, M. L., Steyn-Ross, D. A., Wilson, M. T., & Sleigh, J. W. (2009). Modeling brain activation patterns for the default and cognitive states. *Neuroimage*, 45(2), 298-311.

Stipacek, A., Grabner, R. H., Neuper, C., Fink, A., & Neubauer, A. C. (2003). Sensitivity of human EEG alpha band desynchronization to different working memory components and increasing levels of memory load. *Neurosci Lett*, 353(3), 193-196.

Straube, T., Glauer, M., Dilger, S., Mentzel, H. J., & Miltner, W. H. (2006). Effects of cognitive-behavioral therapy on brain activation in specific phobia. *Neuroimage*, 29(1), 125-135.

Straube, T., & Miltner, W. H. (2011). Attention to aversive emotion and specific activation of the right insula and right somatosensory cortex. *Neuroimage*, 54(3), 2534-2538.

Strohle, A., Stoy, M., Wrase, J., Schwarzer, S., Schlagenhauf, F., Huss, M., et al. (2008). Reward anticipation and outcomes in adult males with attention-deficit/hyperactivity disorder. *Neuroimage*, 39(3), 966-972.

Struve, F. A., Manno, B. R., Kemp, P., Patrick, G., & Manno, J. E. (2003). Acute marihuana (THC) exposure produces a "transient" topographic quantitative EEG profile identical to the "persistent" profile seen in chronic heavy users. *Clin Electroencephalogr*, 34(2), 75-83.

Struve, F. A., Patrick, G., Straumanis, J. J., Fitz-Gerald, M. J., & Manno, J. (1998). Possible EEG sequelae of very long duration marihuana use: pilot findings from topographic quantitative EEG analyses of subjects with 15 to 24 years of cumulative daily exposure to THC. *Clin Electroencephalogr*, 29(1), 31-36.

Struve, F. A., Straumanis, J. J., Patrick, G., & Price, L. (1989). Topographic mapping of quantitative EEG variables in chronic heavy marihuana users: empirical findings with psychiatric patients. *Clin Electroencephalogr*, 20(1), 6-23.

Sumich, A., Matsudaira, T., Gow, R. V., Ibrahimovic, A., Ghebremeskel, K., Crawford, M., et al. (2009). Resting state electroencephalographic correlates with red cell long-chain fatty acids, memory performance and age in adolescent boys with attention deficit hyperactivity disorder. *Neuropharmacology*, 57(7-8), 708-714.

Swartwood, J. N., Swartwood, M. O., Lubar, J. F., & Timmermann, D. L. (2003). EEG differences in ADHD-combined type during baseline and cognitive tasks. *Pediatr Neurol, 28*(3), 199-204.

Takahashi, T., Yücel, M., Lorenzetti, V., Tanino, R., Whittle, S., Suzuki, M., et al. Volumetric MRI study of the insular cortex in individuals with current and past major depression. *Journal of Affective Disorders, 121*(3), 231-238.

Talairach J, T. P. (1988). *Co-planar Stereotaxic Atlas of the Human Brain: 3-Dimensional Proportional System - an Approach to Cerebral Imaging.* New York: Thieme Medical Publishers.

Talairach, J. T., P (1988). *Co-planar Stereoaxic Atlas of the Human Brain.* New York: Theme Medical Publishers.

Tamm, L., Menon, V., & Reiss, A. L. (2006). Parietal attentional system aberrations during target detection in adolescents with attention deficit hyperactivity disorder: event-related fMRI evidence. *Am J Psychiatry, 163*(6), 1033-1043.

Tanaka, K. (1997). Mechanisms of visual object recognition: monkey and human studies. *Curr Opin Neurobiol, 7*(4), 523-529.

Taylor, S. E., Burklund, L. J., Eisenberger, N. I., Lehman, B. J., Hilmert, C. J., & Lieberman, M. D. (2008). Neural bases of moderation of cortisol stress responses by psychosocial resources. *J Pers Soc Psychol, 95*(1), 197-211.

Tedrus, G. M., Fonseca, L. C., Tonelotto, J. M., Costa, R. M., & Chiodi, M. G. (2006). Benign childhood epilepsy with centro-temporal spikes: quantitative EEG and the Wechsler intelligence scale for children (WISC-III). *Clin EEG Neurosci, 37*(3), 193-197.

Teicher, M. H. (2002). Scars that won't heal: the neurobiology of child abuse. *Sci Am, 286*(3), 68-75.

Teicher, M. H., Glod, C. A., Surrey, J., & Swett, C., Jr. (1993). Early childhood abuse and limbic system ratings in adult psychiatric outpatients. J *Neuropsychiatry Clin Neurosci, 5*(3), 301-306.

Teicher, M. H., Samson, J. A., Polcari, A., & Andersen, S. L. (2009). Length of time between onset of childhood sexual abuse and emergence of depression in a young adult sample: a retrospective clinical report. *J Clin Psychiatry, 70*(5), 684-691.

Teicher, M. H., Samson, J. A., Sheu, Y. S., Polcari, A., & McGreenery, C. E. (2010). Hurtful words: association of exposure to peer verbal abuse with elevated psychiatric symptom scores and corpus callosum abnormalities. *Am J Psychiatry, 167*(12), 1464-1471.

Teyler, T. J. (1989). Comparative aspects of hippocampal and neocortical long-term potentiation. *J Neurosci Methods, 28*(1-2), 101-108.

Thatcher, R. W., Biver, C. J., & North, D. M. (2003). Quantitative EEG and the Frye and Daubert standards of admissibility. *Clin Electroencephalogr, 34*(2), 39-53.

Thatcher, R. W., North, D., & Biver, C. (2005a). EEG and intelligence: relations between EEG coherence, EEG phase delay and power. *Clin Neurophysiol, 116*(9), 2129-2141.

Thatcher, R. W., North, D., & Biver, C. (2005b). Evaluation and validity of a LORETA normative EEG database. *Clin EEG Neurosci*, 36(2), 116-122.

Thatcher, R. W., North, D., & Biver, C. (2005c). Parametric vs. non-parametric statistics of low resolution electromagnetic tomography (LORETA). *Clin EEG Neurosci*, 36(1), 1-8.

Thatcher, R. W., North, D., & Biver, C. (2007). Intelligence and EEG current density using low-resolution electromagnetic tomography (LORETA). *Hum Brain Mapp*, 28(2), 118-133.

Thatcher, R. W., North, D. M., & Biver, C. J. (2008). Intelligence and EEG phase reset: a two compartmental model of phase shift and lock. *Neuroimage,* 42(4), 1639-1653.

Thibodeau, R., Jorgensen, R. S., & Kim, S. (2006). Depression, anxiety, and resting frontal EEG asymmetry: a meta-analytic review. *J Abnorm Psychol*, 115(4), 715-729.

Thornton, K. E. (1995). On the Nature of Artifacting the qEEG. *Journal of Neurotherapy,* 1(3), 32-39.

Thornton, L. M., & Andersen, B. L. (2006). Psychoneuroimmunology examined: The role of subjective stress. *Cellscience*, 2(4), nihpa49913.

Tian, L., Jiang, T., Wang, Y., Zang, Y., He, Y., Liang, M., et al. (2006). Altered resting-state functional connectivity patterns of anterior cingulate cortex in adolescents with attention deficit hyperactivity disorder. *Neurosci Lett*, 400(1-2), 39-43.

Timmermann, D. L., Lubar, J. F., Rasey, H. W., & Frederick, J. A. (1999). Effects of 20-min audio-visual stimulation (AVS) at dominant alpha frequency and twice dominant alpha frequency on the cortical EEG. *Int J Psychophysiol,* 32(1), 55-61.

Tislerova, B., Brunovsky, M., Horacek, J., Novak, T., Kopecek, M., Mohr, P., et al. (2008). LORETA functional imaging in antipsychotic-naive and olanzapine-, clozapine- and risperidone-treated patients with schizophrenia. *Neuropsychobiology*, 58(1), 1-10.

Tomarken, A. J., Davidson, R. J., & Henriques, J. B. (1990). Resting frontal brain asymmetry predicts affective responses to films. *J Pers Soc Psychol,* 59(4), 791-801.

Toplak, M. E., Connors, L., Shuster, J., Knezevic, B., & Parks, S. (2008). Review of cognitive, cognitive-behavioral, and neural-based interventions for Attention-Deficit/Hyperactivity Disorder (ADHD). *Clin Psychol Rev*, 28(5), 801-823.

Toro, C., & Deakin, J. F. (2005). NMDA receptor subunit NRI and postsynaptic protein PSD-95 in hippocampus and orbitofrontal cortex in schizophrenia and mood disorder. *Schizophr Res*, 80(2-3), 323-330.

Toro, C. T., Hallak, J. E., Dunham, J. S., & Deakin, J. F. (2006). Glial fibrillary acidic protein and glutamine synthetase in subregions of prefrontal cortex in schizophrenia and mood disorder. *Neurosci Lett*, 404(3), 276-281.

Towle, V. L., Bolanos, J., Suarez, D., Tan, K., Grzeszczuk, R., Levin, D. N., et al. (1993). The spatial location of EEG electrodes: locating the best-fitting sphere relative to cortical anatomy. *Electroencephalogr Clin Neurophysiol*, 86(1), 1-6.

Tricomi, E. M., Delgado, M. R., & Fiez, J. A. (2004). Modulation of caudate activity by action contingency. Neuron, 41(2), 281-292.

Triffleman, E., Carroll, K., & Kellogg, S. (1999). Substance dependence posttraumatic stress disorder therapy. An integrated cognitive-behavioral approach. *J Subst Abuse Treat*, 17(1-2), 3-14.

Uddin, L. Q., Kaplan, J. T., Molnar-Szakacs, I., Zaidel, E., & Iacoboni, M. (2005). Self-face recognition activates a frontoparietal "mirror" network in the right hemisphere: an event-related fMRI study. *Neuroimage*, 25(3), 926-935.

Vaden, K. I., Piquado, T., & Hickok, G. (2011). Sublexical Properties of Spoken Words Modulate Activity in Broca's Area but Not Superior Temporal Cortex: Implications for Models of Speech Recognition. *J Cogn Neurosci*. 23:2665-2674

Valdes-Hernandez, P. A., Ojeda-Gonzalez, A., Martinez-Montes, E., Lage-Castellanos, A., Virues-Alba, T., Valdes-Urrutia, L., et al. (2010). White matter architecture rather than cortical surface area correlates with the EEG alpha rhythm. *Neuroimage*, 49(3), 2328-2339.

van Reekum, C. M., Urry, H. L., Johnstone, T., Thurow, M. E., Frye, C. J., Jackson, C. A., et al. (2007). Individual differences in amygdala and ventromedial prefrontal cortex activity are associated with evaluation speed and psychological well-being. *J Cogn Neurosci*, 19(2), 237-248.

Vance, A., Silk, T. J., Casey, M., Rinehart, N. J., Bradshaw, J. L., Bellgrove, M. A., et al. (2007). Right parietal dysfunction in children with attention deficit hyperactivity disorder, combined type: a functional MRI study. *Mol Psychiatry*, 12(9), 826-832, 793.

Venneman, S., Leuchter, A., Bartzokis, G., Beckson, M., Simon, S. L., Schaefer, M., et al. (2006). Variation in neurophysiological function and evidence of quantitative electroencephalogram discordance: predicting cocaine-dependent treatment attrition. *J Neuropsychiatry Clin Neurosci,* 18(2), 208-216.

Vitacco, D., Brandeis, D., Pascual-Marqui, R., & Martin, E. (2002). Correspondence of event-related potential tomography and functional magnetic resonance imaging during language processing. *Hum Brain Mapp*, 17(1), 4-12.

Vogeley, K., & Fink, G. R. (2003). Neural correlates of the first-person-perspective. T*rends Cogn Sci*, 7(1), 38-42.

Vogt, B. A., Derbyshire, S., & Jones, A. K. (1996). Pain processing in four regions of human cingulate cortex localized with co-registered PET and MR imaging. *Eur J Neurosci,* 8(7), 1461-1473.

Vogt, B. A., Finch, D. M., & Olson, C. R. (1992). Functional heterogeneity in cingulate cortex: the anterior executive and posterior evaluative regions. *Cereb Cortex*, 2(6), 435-443.

Vogt, B. A., Nimchinsky, E. A., Vogt, L. J., & Hof, P. R. (1995). Human cingulate cortex: surface features, flat maps, and cytoarchitecture. *J Comp Neurol*, 359(3), 490-506.

Vogt, B. A., Wiley, R. G., & Jensen, E. L. (1995). Localization of Mu and delta opioid receptors to anterior cingulate afferents and projection neurons and input/output model of Mu regulation. *Exp Neurol,* 135(2), 83-92.

Vogt, F., Klimesch, W., & Doppelmayr, M. (1998). High-frequency components in the alpha band and memory performance. *J Clin Neurophysiol,* 15(2), 167-172.

Volkow, N. D., Wang, G. J., Fowler, J. S., Logan, J., Jayne, M., Franceschi, D., et al. (2002). "Nonhedonic" food motivation in humans involves dopamine in the dorsal striatum and methylphenidate amplifies this effect. *Synapse,* 44(3), 175-180.

Volkow, N. D., Wang, G. J., Kollins, S. H., Wigal, T. L., Newcorn, J. H., Telang, F., et al. (2009). Evaluating dopamine reward pathway in ADHD: clinical implications. *JAMA,* 302(10), 1084-1091.

Volz, K. G., Schubotz, R. I., & von Cramon, D. Y. (2005). Variants of uncertainty in decision-making and their neural correlates. *Brain Res Bull,* 67(5), 403-412.

Wackerly, D. D., Mendenhall, III, W., Scheaffer, R.L. (2002). *Mathematical Statistics with Applications (Sixth ed.).* Pacific Grove: Duxbury.

Wagner, M., Fuchs, M., & Kastner, J. (2004). Evaluation of sLORETA in the presence of noise and multiple sources. *Brain Topogr,* 16(4), 277-280.

Wallstrom, G. L., Kass, R. E., Miller, A., Cohn, J. F., & Fox, N. A. (2004). Automatic correction of ocular artifacts in the EEG: a comparison of regression-based and component-based methods. *Int J Psychophysiol,* 53(2), 105-119.

Walton, M. E., Croxson, P. L., Behrens, T. E., Kennerley, S. W., & Rushworth, M. F. (2007). Adaptive decision making and value in the anterior cingulate cortex. *Neuroimage,* 36 Suppl 2, T142-154.

Wang, G. J., Volkow, N. D., & Fowler, J. S. (2002). The role of dopamine in motivation for food in humans: implications for obesity. *Expert Opin Ther Targets,* 6(5), 601-609.

Wang, J., Korczykowski, M., Rao, H., Fan, Y., Pluta, J., Gur, R. C., et al. (2007). Gender difference in neural response to psychological stress. *Soc Cogn Affect Neurosci,* 2(3), 227-239.

Wang, J., Rao, H., Wetmore, G. S., Furlan, P. M., Korczykowski, M., Dinges, D. F., et al. (2005). Perfusion functional MRI reveals cerebral blood flow pattern under psychological stress. *Proc Natl Acad Sci U S A,* 102(49), 17804-17809.

Watamura, S. E., Donzella, B., Alwin, J., & Gunnar, M. R. (2003). Morning-to-afternoon increases in cortisol concentrations for infants and toddlers at child care: age differences and behavioral correlates. *Child Dev,* 74(4), 1006-1020.

Weiskopf, N., Mathiak, K., Bock, S. W., Scharnowski, F., Veit, R., Grodd, W., et al. (2004). Principles of a brain-computer interface (BCI) based on real-time functional magnetic resonance imaging (fMRI). *IEEE Trans Biomed Eng,* 51(6), 966-970.

Weiskopf, N., Scharnowski, F., Veit, R., Goebel, R., Birbaumer, N., & Mathiak, K. (2004). Self-regulation of local brain activity using real-time functional magnetic resonance imaging (fMRI). *J Physiol Paris*, 98(4-6), 357-373.

Weissman, D. H., Roberts, K. C., Visscher, K. M., & Woldorff, M. G. (2006). The neural bases of momentary lapses in attention. *Nat Neurosci*, 9(7), 971-978.

Wender, P. H. (1995). *Attention-deficit hyperactivity disorder in adults*. New York: Oxford University Press.

Werkle-Bergner, M., Muller, V., Li, S. C., & Lindenberger, U. (2006). Cortical EEG correlates of successful memory encoding: implications for lifespan comparisons. *Neurosci Biobehav Rev,* 30(6), 839-854.

Westermeyer, J., Kopka, S., & Nugent, S. (1997). Course and severity of substance abuse among patients with comorbid major depression. *Am J Addict*, 6(4), 284-292.

Whalen, P. J., Bush, G., McNally, R. J., Wilhelm, S., McInerney, S. C., Jenike, M. A., et al. (1998). The emotional counting Stroop paradigm: a functional magnetic resonance imaging probe of the anterior cingulate affective division. *Biol Psychiatry,* 44(12), 1219-1228.

White, B. R., Snyder, A. Z., Cohen, A. L., Petersen, S. E., Raichle, M. E., Schlaggar, B. L., et al. (2009). Resting-state functional connectivity in the human brain revealed with diffuse optical tomography. *Neuroimage*, 47(Supplement 1), S-163.

White, J. A., Banks, M. I., Pearce, R. A., & Kopell, N. J. (2000). Networks of interneurons with fast and slow gamma-aminobutyric acid type A (GABAA) kinetics provide substrate for mixed gamma-theta rhythm. *Proc Natl Acad Sci U S A*, 97(14), 8128-8133.

Wickens, J. R., Reynolds, J. N., & Hyland, B. I. (2003). Neural mechanisms of reward-related motor learning. *Curr Opin Neurobiol*, 13(6), 685-690.

Wilens, T. E., Biederman, J., & Mick, E. (1998). Does ADHD affect the course of substance abuse? Findings from a sample of adults with and without ADHD. *Am J Addict,* 7(2), 156-163.

Willis, W. G., & Weiler, M. D. (2005). Neural substrates of childhood attention-deficit/hyperactivity disorder: electroencephalographic and magnetic resonance imaging evidence. *Dev Neuropsychol,* 27(1), 135-182.

Winterer, G., Mahlberg, R., Smolka, M. N., Samochowiec, J., Ziller, M., Rommelspacher, H. P., et al. (2003). Association analysis of exonic variants of the GABA(B)-receptor gene and alpha electroencephalogram voltage in normal subjects and alcohol-dependent patients. *Behav Genet*, 33(1), 7-15.

Winterer, G., Ziller, M., Kloppel, B., Heinz, A., Schmidt, L. G., & Herrmann, W. M. (1998). Analysis of quantitative EEG with artificial neural networks and discriminant analysis--a methodological comparison. *Neuropsychobiology*, 37(1), 41-48.

Wise, B. K., Cuffe, S. P., & Fischer, T. (2001). Dual diagnosis and successful participation of adolescents in substance abuse treatment. *J Subst Abuse Treat*, 21(3), 161-165.

Wise, R. A. (2004). Dopamine, learning and motivation. *Nat Rev Neurosci,* 5(6), 483-494.

Woodruff-Pak, D. S., & Gould, T. J. (2002). Neuronal nicotinic acetylcholine receptors: involvement in Alzheimer's disease and schizophrenia. *Behav Cogn Neurosci Rev,* 1(1), 5-20.

Woodward, D. J., Chang, J. Y., Janak, P., Azarov, A., & Anstrom, K. (1999). Mesolimbic neuronal activity across behavioral states. *Ann N Y Acad Sci,* 877, 91-112.

Worrell, G. A., Lagerlund, T. D., Sharbrough, F. W., Brinkmann, B. H., Busacker, N. E., Cicora, K. M., et al. (2000). Localization of the epileptic focus by low-resolution electromagnetic tomography in patients with a lesion demonstrated by MRI. *Brain Topogr,* 12(4), 273-282.

Yang, T. T., Simmons, A. N., Matthews, S. C., Tapert, S. F., Bischoff-Grethe, A., Frank, G. K., et al. (2007). Increased amygdala activation is related to heart rate during emotion processing in adolescent subjects. *Neurosci Lett,* 428(2-3), 109-114.

Yao, Z., Wang, L., Lu, Q., Liu, H., & Teng, G. (2009). Regional homogeneity in depression and its relationship with separate depressive symptom clusters: A resting-state fMRI study. *Journal of Affective Disorders,* 115(3), 430-438.

Yerys, B. E., Jankowski, K. F., Shook, D., Rosenberger, L. R., Barnes, K. A., Berl, M. M., et al. (2009). The fMRI success rate of children and adolescents: typical development, epilepsy, attention deficit/hyperactivity disorder, and autism spectrum disorders. *Hum Brain Mapp,* 30(10), 3426-3435.

Yordanova, J., & Kolev, V. (1997). Developmental changes in the event-related EEG theta response and P300. *Electroencephalogr Clin Neurophysiol,* 104(5), 418-430.

Young, J. (1990). *Cognitive therapy for personality disorders: A schema-focused approach.* Sarasota: Professional Resource Press.

Zametkin, A. J., Nordahl, T. E., Gross, M., King, A. C., Semple, W. E., Rumsey, J., et al. (1990). Cerebral glucose metabolism in adults with hyperactivity of childhood onset. *N Engl J Med,* 323(20), 1361-1366.

Zang, Y. F., Jin, Z., Weng, X. C., Zhang, L., Zeng, Y. W., Yang, L., et al. (2005). Functional MRI in attention-deficit hyperactivity disorder: evidence for hypofrontality. *Brain Dev,* 27(8), 544-550.

Zhang, Z., Jiao, Y. Y., & Sun, Q. Q. (2011). Developmental maturation of excitation and inhibition balance in principal neurons across four layers of somatosensory cortex. *Neuroscience,* 174, 10-25.

Zhou, Y., Dougherty, J. H., Jr., Hubner, K. F., Bai, B., Cannon, R. L., & Hutson, R. K. (2008). Abnormal connectivity in the posterior cingulate and hippocampus in early Alzheimer's disease and mild cognitive impairment. *Alzheimers Dement,* 4(4), 265-270.

Zola-Morgan, S., & Squire, L. R. (1985). Medial temporal lesions in monkeys impair memory on a variety of tasks sensitive to human amnesia. *Behav Neurosci,* 99(1), 22-34.

Zola-Morgan, S., Squire, L. R., & Amaral, D. G. (1986). Human amnesia and the medial temporal region: enduring memory impairment following a bilateral lesion limited to field CA1 of the hippocampus. *J Neurosci,* 6(10), 2950-2967.

Zola-Morgan, S., Squire, L. R., Amaral, D. G., & Suzuki, W. A. (1989). Lesions of perirhinal and parahippocampal cortex that spare the amygdala and hippocampal formation produce severe memory impairment. *J Neurosci,* 9(12), 4355-4370.

Zola-Morgan, S., Squire, L. R., Rempel, N. L., Clower, R. P., & Amaral, D. G. (1992). Enduring memory impairment in monkeys after ischemic damage to the hippocampus. *J Neurosci,* 12(7), 2582-2596.

Zschocke, S., Speckmann, E. (Ed.). (2000). *Basic Mechanisms of the EEG.* Boston: Birkhäuser

Zumsteg, D., Andrade, D. M., & Wennberg, R. A. (2006). Source localization of small sharp spikes: low resolution electromagnetic tomography (LORETA) reveals two distinct cortical sources. *Clin Neurophysiol,* 117(6), 1380-1387.

Zumsteg, D., Wennberg, R. A., Treyer, V., Buck, A., & Wieser, H. G. (2005). H2(15)O or 13NH3 PET and electromagnetic tomography (LORETA) during partial status epilepticus. *Neurology,* 65(10), 1657-1660.

CPSIA information can be obtained
at www.ICGtesting.com
Printed in the USA
LVIC080057050912
297236LV00002BA

* 9 7 8 0 9 8 2 7 4 9 8 1 4 *